MW01282629

The Best of Wits End

The Best of Wits End

Medical Humor at Its Brainiest

Harold J. Ellner, M.D.

Copyright © 2008 by Harold J. Ellner, M.D.

Cover illustration by Lou Myers.

Library of Congress Control Number: 2007909365
ISBN: Hardcover   978-1-4363-0616-4
                   Softcover   978-1-4363-0615-7

All rights reserved. No part of this book may be reproduced or transmitted in any form
or by any means, electronic or mechanical, including photocopying, recording, or by
any information storage and retrieval system, without permission in writing from the
copyright owner.

This book was printed in the United States of America.

To order additional copies of this book, contact:
Xlibris Corporation
1-888-795-4274
www.Xlibris.com
Orders@Xlibris.com
39222

CONTENTS

Dedication

To founder Norton Bramesco, Dr. Joseph F.J. Curi, Dr. Meyer Hodes, and all those whose goodness and joyful humor shall survive them interminably.

Gratitude goes to Ed Wetschler, editor par excellence, for his patience and expertise.

For the twenty-five years ending in 2004, there appeared, at the terminal page of a magazine devoted to physicians' pastimes and interests, a department called Wits End. It was the creation of Norton Bramesco, a career writer of pharmaceutical advertising copy. He sold the magazine's officers on the concept of a monthly contest to tap the lode of wit in medical minds. And tap it, it did. From its inception, the column filled some needs:

- It invoked formidable satirical talent.
- Under the cloak of humor, there surfaced creative expressions of criticism directed at latter-day constraints on medical practice.
- It evoked hilarity.
- Above all, it was the only department of the nonclinical publication that allowed for the camaraderie of doctors as doctors. Otherwise, they were merely readers or, occasionally, writers of letters to the editor.

Nonphysicians shared in this, offering numerous contributions before it became policy to limit entries to MDs and DOs. Such participation demonstrated that the activity was not so arcane as to appeal only to doctors. Most of the entries in this volume are, in fact, understandable to the laity.

Norton Bramesco used the pseudonym "Daedalus." He accompanied each page with a lively and engaging banter. When a fatal illness took him at far too early an age, his successor (HJE) unsurprisingly chose "Icarus" as a pen name.

Contestants from every state poured in their efforts. Some did so with regularity. Others appeared brilliantly albeit briefly. Between these extremes were many degrees of intermittent participation. The contests were ordained each to have a medical twist, as the reader will readily see. Moreover, of the 180-odd challenges in the era of Icarus, no two were the same. Entrants grew to be prepared for a surprise each time. Seemingly, they had no trouble adjusting. The culled results that follow represent a fraction of the wit and humor that rained in on the magazine's office. Multiple entries were, perforce, pared to the adjudged best one of any submitted list.

The purpose of setting down the best of the last fifteen years of the span of Wits End is an effort to prevent the disappearance into oblivion of the output of the wittiest medical minds imaginable.

Some of the more X-rated submissions, not printable during the life of the series, appear, apocryphally, at the end of the collection.

Enjoy.

Harold "Icarus" J. Ellner, MD

O GIVE ME A HOME

ASSIGNMENT:
Select an appropriately named community for the golden years of a retired practitioner.

EXAMPLES:
Neurologist—Las Vagus, NE
Podiatrist—Frankfoot, Germany
Endocrinologist—Glandover, MD
Pulmonologist—The Bronchs, NY

ENTRIES:
Nephrologist—Salt Leak City, UT

Bernadine Paulshock, MD, Wilmington, DE

Psychiatrist—Amitypill, LI

Meyer Hodes, MD, Oceanside, NY

Otolaryngologist—Buenos Nares, Argentina

Michael Ichniowski, MD, Lutherville, MD

Psychiatrist—Jungstown, OH

Morey Filler, MD, San Francisco, CA

Dental Surgeon—Gnashville, TN

Joan Levin, Jacksonville, FL

Obstetrician (breech deliveries)—Rearborn, MI

Steven Drosman, MD, San Diego, CA

Diabetologist—Sweetwater, TN

T. E. Cummings, MD, Rockmart, GA

Trauma Surgeon—Woundsockett, RI

Jay Schinfeld, MD, Melrose Park, PA

Urologist—Lake Flaccid, NY

Richard R. Morris, MD, Harrison, OH

Urologist—Pisscataway, NJ

Howard M. Graubard, MD, Pembroke Pines, FL

OPERATIC OPERATIONS

ASSIGNMENT:
Name a musical opus playable at a surgical procedure.

EXAMPLES:
"O Sole Mio"—Plantar wart removal

"The Lost C(h)ord"—Vasectomy

"I've Got You Under My Skin"—Foreign body extraction

ENTRIES:
"The Last Time I Saw Paris"—Plaster cast removal
Susan R. Owen, RN, Findlay, OH

"Both Sides Now"—Bilateral hernia repair
Mark Williams, MD, Riverside, CA

"Till We Meet Again"—Vasectomy repair
Doris Fletcher, Kendall Park, NJ

"Looking for Love in All the Wrong Places"—Removal of venereal warts
Robert L. Hillery, MD, Findlay, OH

Overture to Fals(e)taff—Penile implant
Paul D. Fuchs, MD, Bronx, NY

"Baby, It's Cold Outside"—Cesarean section
J. Patrick Evans, Savannah, GA

"Toot Toot Tootsie, Goodbye"—Amputation of toe
Kenneth A. Deitcher, MD, Albany, NY

Mahler's Resurrection Symphony—Cardiac resuscitation
Charles G. Eschenburg, MD, Delray Beach, FL

"Stop! In the Name of Love"—Tubal ligation
John F. Bonomo, MD, Chatham, NJ

"I Left My Heart in San Francisco"—Transplant donor
James C. Farley, MD, Laflin, PA

IATRIC IAMBS

ASSIGNMENT:
Add a medical second line to the first line of a well-known poem.

EXAMPLES:
The outlook wasn't brilliant for the Mudville nine that day,
Their star was hit by pitcher in the median raphè.

When lilacs last in the dooryard bloom'd,
Antihistamine sales zoomed.

Abou Ben Adhem (may his tribe increase!)
Ruled he that all vasectomies cease.

ENTRIES:
There was a crooked man and he walked a crooked mile,
He's had kyphoscoliosis ever since he was a chil'.

Doris E. Fletcher, Kendall Park, NJ

Wee, sleekit, cow'rin, tim'rous beastie
Be ye virus, bacterium, or yeastie?

Ivan M. Safonoff, MD, New York City, NY

Wynken, Blynken, and Nod one night
Gave their neurologist quite a fright.

Suzanne E. Mahan, MD, Pueblo, CO

Fifteen men on the dead man's chest,
Run for the crash cart and bring back the rest.

Samuel A. Brewton, Jr., MD, Thomaston, GA

Who shall decide when doctors disagree?
The pathologist, most probably.

Stanley Ostern, MD, Santa Barbara, CA

Hickory, Dickory, Doc!
Your lab mouse is in shock.

D. Stanley Hartness, MD, Kosciusco, MS

Gather ye rosebuds while ye may,
I just got the report on your X-ray.

Arthur S. Verdusca, MD, Morristown, NJ

While winds frae off Ben Lomond blaw,
Colds come, then bills without a flaw.

Christina M. Martan, Carson, GA

Jenny kiss'd me when we met;
No sign of herpes virus yet.

Arthur L. Kobal, DDS, Covina, CA

A bunch of the boys were whooping it up in the Malamute saloon;
'Til the cops appeared and made them inflate the breathalyzer balloon.

William M. Kane, MD, Hays, KS

Whan that Aprill with his shoures soote,
Allergy patients, hands to nose, salute.

Stuart M. Copperman, MD, Merrick, NY

LITERARY LAUNDERINGS

ASSIGNMENT:

In a double-entendre challenge, create a medical meaning to a book title.

EXAMPLES:

Closing the Ring—Hernia repairs down through the ages.

The Pride of the Yankees—Self-assertion among the newly edentulous.

The Boston Strangler—The Massachusetts Medicare Mangle Mastermind

ENTRIES:

Lonesome Dove—Memoirs of the last bar of soap at the newborn nursery scrub sink.

Russell J. Cox, MD, Gastonia, NC

Advise and Consent—Legal aspects of preparing today's surgical patients.

Samuel A. Brewton, MD, Thomaston, GA

Blue Highways—The diagnosis and management of varicose veins.

Doris E. Fletcher, Kendall Park, NJ

The Rise and Fall of the Great Powers—The life and times of Don Juan from puberty to impotency.

Ray L. Landreneau, MD, Mobile, AL

The Turn of the Screw—A young orthopedist struggles to make ends meet.

Ivan M. Safonoff, MD, NYC, NY

The Hunt for Red October—Doctor, am I pregnant?

Richard Schuldenfrei, MD, N. Andover, MA

Islands in the Stream—A serious urological problem.

J. Patrick Evans, MD, Savannah, GA

Stand and Deliver—An obstetrician and his hemorrhoids.

Harrison C. Fisher, MD, Lahaina, Maui, HI

Clear and Present Danger—Chronicles the meteoric rise of the number of lawyers in the malpractice industry.

Richard H. Morris, MD, Harrison, OH

Great Expectations—Ultrasound as predictor of a normal fetus

Grafton C. Fanney, Jr., MD, Euclid, OH

Finnegan's Wake—Help for the insomniac.

Stephen L. Kaufman, MD, San Francisco CA

MOMENTS OF GREAT MOMENT

ASSIGNMENT:

When ether was first given, the anesthetist's immortal words were, "Your patient is ready, Doctor." Paraphrase it as if some well-known person were giving the anesthesia.

EXAMPLES:

ROBERT BURNS: "'Tis a bricht licht shinin' on the sicht. Wield yere ane wee knife, laddie."

CLINT EASTWOOD: "Come on. Make his day. Operate."

P. G. WODEHOUSE: "I say, dash it all, time to set the old lemon a-throbbing and cluster about this sleeping bloke."

ENTRIES:

WINSTON CHURCHILL: "We shall not fail. We shall clamp each bleeder. We shall defend the pulse with growing confidence, whatever the cost may be. We shall monitor the air, control the sea of blood, bind the lacerated body. Carry on, surgeon: Dread naught. Godspeed!"

Donald Barkan, MD, Swampscott, MA

BOGUS BORDER GUARD from *The Treasure of Sierra Madre*: "Gas? Gas? We don't need no stinkin' gas; cut the gringo!"

Richard A. Mingione, MD, Atlantic City, NJ

WILLIAM SHAKESPEARE: "His sleep is not so peaceful as a forest stream or so untroubled as a babe at breast, but 'tis deep enough, 'twill serve. Lay on, my dear good Lord."

Richard H. Johnson, MD, Atlanta, GA
Meyer B. Hodes, MD, Oceanside, NY

MELVIN BELLI: "Make that incision, I dare you."

M. David Lauter, MD, York, ME

RHETT BUTLER: "Yes, I know the patient's abdomen is not relaxed, but frankly, my dear, I don't give a damn."

> Samuel A Brewton, MD, Thomaston, GA
> Ken Deitcher, MD, Albany, NY

NATHAN HALE: "I regret that I have but one hour for you to complete this case."

> Karen Hulett, MD, Jackson, MS

JACK BENNY: "Cut that out!"

> Charles L. Aumiller, MD, Boulder, CO

MAE WEST: "Why don't you come up and operate sometime, big boy?"

> Marc S. Williams, MD, Riverside, CA

SUPER GROUPERS

ASSIGNMENT:
Create a catch name for a specialty clinic

EXAMPLES:
Rheummates—Arthritis clinic
The Gang of Formula—Pediatric group
The Armed Surfaces—Dermatologists

ENTRIES:
Natal Alliance—Obstetricians

Edward M. Sessa, MD, Schenectady, NY

The Ovary Hill Gang—OB-GYN clinic

Angela Poe, LPN, James B. Ball, MD, Bettsville, OH

Urine Good Hands Group—Nephrology group

B. J. Cochrane, MD, Watertown, WI

Final Four—Forensic pathology group

Lawrence K. Harris, MD, Reading, PA

Suitcases—Professional witness group

Charles L. Aumiller, MD, Boulder, CO

Faternity Brothers—Bariatricians

Donald Stoltz, DO, Philadelphia, PA

Tick Docs—Lyme disease experts

Alan R. La Reau, MD, Kalamazoo, MI

The Patients' Wait Loss Center—Minor emergency walk-in clinic

Russell J. Cox, MD, Gastonia, NC

Truss Busters—Group of hernia surgeons

Evelyn L. Weissman, MD, Malone, NY

The Stork Exchange—A perinatal practice

Suzanne E. Mahan, MD, Pueblo, CO

Wind-O-Pain—Pulmonology

Karl Brandspigel, MD, Elizabeth City, NC

Cankers Away!—Dermatologists

Renee Katz, Bronx, NY

The Meta Mucils—A geriatric group

Marc Gordon, Bronx, NY

Strange Bedfellows—Sex therapists

Steven G. Manikas, DO, Ann Arbor, MI

And the conglomerated urologists' contributions, per Michael H. Phillips, MD, Washington, DC, and William J. Somers, MD, Nassawadox, VA, to wit, the Erector Set, the Stream Team, the Rod Squad—All urology groups

THE 800 CLUB

ASSIGNMENT:
Select a seven-digit 800 number appropriate to a type of practice.

EXAMPLES:
Two-physician partnership: 1-800-PARADOX
Neurosurgeon: 1-800-CRANIUM
Acupuncturist: 1-800-PRIKKEM

ENTRIES:
Echo-imaging technician: 1-800-180080
> Donald Barkan, MD, Swampscott, MA

Psychiatrist-geneticist: 1-800-CYCLONE
> Edgar A. Calvelo, MD, Napa, CA

Nutritionist: 1-800-URWATU8
> Marie Dunford, RD, Kingsburg, CA

Proctosigmoidoscopist: 1-800-WATTSUP
> J. R. Sevenich, MD, Stevens Point, WI

Liposuctionist: 1-800-SLURPIT
> William M. Kane, MD, Hays, KS

Impotence clinic: 1-800-PRIAPIC
> Stephen H. Mintz, MD, Syracuse, NY

Gynecologist: 1-800-DRDANDC
> Brent N. Davidson, MD, West Bloomfield, MI

Fertility specialists: 1-800-EGGDROP
> James M. Friedman, MD, Fort Worth, TX

Substance abuse center: 1-800-UR2HIGH
> Melvin J. Breite, MD, Bayside, NY

Psychiatrist: 1-800-TIMESUP

Evan M Ginsberg, MD, Hamden, CT

Gynecologist: 1-800-4XXONLY

Esfand Nawab, MD, Bethesda, MD

Dermatologist: 1-800-ZITSEND

Charles Patterson, RPh, Duncanville, TX

Sperm bank: 1-800-DADDIEO

Patricia Vondrak, Largo, FL

WHAT HAVE YOU DONE FOR HIM LATELY?

ASSIGNMENT:
Contrive a way to repay Santa Claus medically.

EXAMPLES:
Treatment of Rudolph's rhinophyma.
Cleansing of sooty chimney shaft abrasions.
Respiratory therapy for the hypoxia of high flying.

ENTRIES:
A Texas (external) catheter for those long stretches between continents.

Frank Fusco, MD, Shawnee-on-Delaware, PA

Speech therapy for echolalia (Ho! Ho! Ho!).

Morey Filler, MD, San Francisco, CA

Treatment for Nintendinitis developed while delivering video games.

Charles Patterson, RPh, Duncanville, TX

Psychotherapy to relieve constant state of euphoria.

Henry J. Dold, MD, Barrington, IL

Gas relief from milk intolerance.

Michael R. Cohen, MD, Petersburg, VA

Growth hormone therapy for short-statured helpers.

A. R. La Reau, MD, Kalamazoo, MI

Eight flea-and-tick collars, a free Lyme titer, and a season's worth of tetracycline.

Edward M. Sessa, MD, Schenectady, NY

Valium for Santa's severe case of sleigh-lag.

Marc Williams, MD, Moreno Valley, CA

A Cigarrest to be held between teeth, instead of that pipe.

Sue Diamond, Ormond Beach, FL

Audiologic evaluation with fitting of hearing aid for deafness induced by constant jingling of bells.

Meyer B. Hodes, MD, Oceanside, NY

An elf-cloning set to relieve production stress.

Charles G. Eschenburg, MD, Delray Beach, FL

TO FADE AWAY

ASSIGNMENT:
Paraphrase MacArthur's quotation from the song "Old Soldiers Never Die, They Just Fade Away" to apply to elderly medical types.

EXAMPLES:
Old ophthalmologists never die—they just lose contact.
Old gastroenterologists never die—they are just purged.
Old endoscopists never die—they just go down the tube.

ENTRIES:
Old cytologists . . . they just go on to a higher power.

Patricia Hays, MD, Corona Del Mar, CA

Old proctologists . . . reach the end.

Michael R. Cohen, MD, Petersburg, VA

Old neurologists . . . tap out.

Michael J. Zappitelli, MD, Norristown, PA

Old HMO specialists . . . just get de-capitated

Robert Glenn, MD, Little Rock, AR

Old urologists . . . go null and void.

William R. McCurry, MD, Redding, CA

Old geneticists . . . they just return to the gene pool.

Nancy Spates, MD, Lansing, MI

Old geriatricians . . . become the problem instead of the solution.

Carlyn Kline, MD, St. Joseph, MO

Old neurologists . . . just circle the Willis.

Joe Freund, MD, Eldora, IA

Old psychiatrists . . . shrink away.

Charles Nagurka, MD, Los Angeles, CA

Old hematologists . . . recirculate.

William Graves, MD, and Alice Graves, JD,
St. Petersburg, FL

Old cardiac surgeons . . . get bypassed.

Dilip Bharene, MD, New York, NY
Ranjini Kandasamy, MD, Honolulu, HI

DOUBLE SWIFTIES

ASSIGNMENT:
Contrive a medical situation using Tom Swifties in both verb and adverb (or adverbial phrase).

EXAMPLES:
"I asked for a stiff scrub brush," bristled Tom abrasively.

"Ride down to the hospital basement with me," understated Tom condescendingly.

"This is just a small catheter," piped Tom in passing.

ENTRIES:
"The tumor began in the wrist," carped Tom crabbily.

Carlyn M. Kline, MD, St. Joseph, MO

"Lithotripsy is sure expensive," boomed Tom stonily.

William H. Stover, MD, North Bend, OR

"It's only a chest cold," coughed Tom phlegmatically.

Robert R. Johns, MD, Lafayette, LA

"I would like some rubber gloves," snapped Tom offhandedly.

Robert L. Hillery, MD, Findlay, OH

"Move to Arizona," stated Tom dryly.

Renee Katz, Bronx, NY

"It's only gastric reflux," belched Tom acidly.

W. H. Gordon, MD, San Antonio, TX

"We've got to inflate those lungs," bellowed Tom resonantly.

Brian W. Donnelly, MD, Freehold, NJ

"Prepare the patient's favorite dessert," Tom minced piously.

T. Ben Kalman, MD, San Diego, CA

"pHooey on the Henderson-Hasselbalch equation," pHonated pHoebe acidly.

Doris E. Fletcher, Kendall Park, NJ

"Tell the laundry these OR scrubs don't cling anymore," charged Tom ecstatically.

Meyer B. Hodes, MD Oceanside, NY

"Hip prostheses present no problem," articulated Tom and his assistant jointly.

Samuel Brewton, MD, Thomaston, GA

UNHOMEBODIES

ASSIGNMENT:
The traveler's nightmare is to be stricken by illness in a faraway place. Match a foreign place and illness in rhyme.

EXAMPLES:
Dyscrasia in Asia
Edema in Lima
A fistula on the Vistula

ENTRIES:
Ruptured diverticulum on the Janiculum (a hill in Rome)

William E. Somerall, Jr., MD, Birmingham, AL

Mal de mer in Val-d'Isere (or anywhere).

Richard Jonas, MD, Laguna Beach, CA
Dr. Louis DiBacco, Aldan, PA

Tsk-tsk—what she had in Trinidad!

Mona M. Ruwaldt, MD, Syracuse, NY

Tabes dorsalis in Buckingham Palace

Dr. Michael Ichniowski, Lutherville, MD

Torsade de pointes in Paris, France

Peter J. Stahl, MD, Columbia, MO

Montezuma's Revenge at Stonehenge

Doris E. Fletcher, Kendall Park, NJ

Kidney stone along the Rhone

Allan R. La Reau, MD, Kalamazoo, MI

Venereal sore in Ecuador

Donald D. Schrein, MD, Omaha, NE

Catatonia in Macedonia

Arthur S. Verdesca, MD, Morristown, NJ

Celiac sprue at Waterloo

Henry Bianchi, MD, Tucson, AZ

Migraine aura in Bora-Bora

Laurie Bayer, MD, Washington, DC

COUNTRY DOCTOR MUSIC

ASSIGNMENT:
Create a medical song title bearing a bucolic flavor.

EXAMPLES:
"When You Told Me I Was Your Heartthrob, It Was Only an Atrial Fib"
"The Fellers Call Him Arthroscope Because He Can Case Any Joint"
"Your Reflex Bladder Promises Don't Hold No Water with Me"

ENTRIES:
"I've Learned to Love Dementia Now That I Can't Remember You"
Carlyn Kline, MD, St. Joseph, MO

"I Knew She Was an Alcoholic, but I Loved Her Still"
Robert L. Hillery, MD, Findlay, OH

"I'm Just an In-Law on Your Relative Value Scale"
Howard H. Heller, MD, Oak Harbor, WA

"Your Cheatin' Ways Made Coleslaw of My CABG"
Thomas J. Durkin, Jr., MD, Huntington Valley, PA

Stagecoach driver's song: "When You See My Peyronie's, You'll Know I'm Coming Round the Bend"
Gene R. Savelkoul, MD, Belgrade, MN

"If I Told You That You Had a Beautiful Stethoscope, Would You Hold It Against My Heart?"
Joseph B. Szgalsky, MD, Woodbury, NJ

"She May Have Been a Hypochondriac, but Her Memory Malingers On"
David M. Boeckman, OD, Conroe, TX

"Since She Had Her Hysterectomy, There's Womb in Her Life for Me"

Henderson Powell, MD, West Columbia, SC

"It Was Only Diabetes When I Thought She Was Sweet on Me"

Patrick M. Boccagno, MD, Altoona, PA

"Some Broken Hearts Don't Mend, but the Beat Goes On"

Michael J. Zappitelli, DO, Norristown, PA

STAGE WHISPERS

ASSIGNMENT:
Give a play review in the words of a medical specialist.

EXAMPLES:
Gastroenterologist: "A play of great scope, a moving performance."
Orthopedist: "Grossly humerus."
Ophthalmologist: "Never had so much fundus in my life."

ENTRIES:
Pediatrician: "See Dick act. See Jane act. Act, Spot, act. Run theatergoers, run."

Stuart M. Copperman, MD, Merrick, NY

Pulmonologist: "Acute thespitory distress."

Jonathan S. Ehrlich, MD, Atlanta, GA

Family practitioner: "The Chorea(n)-based play was done with much fever . . . I could feel my heart . . . A murmur developed into a rash of applause, and soon the joint swelled into an ovation."

Richard P. Day, MD, Sioux Falls, SD

Proctologist: "Piles of fun, but a painful performance in the end."

Jeffrey M. Simon, MD, San Pedro, CA

Gastroenterologist: "A 'gas'; rumblings of greatness, waves of laughter, easy to swallow."

H. Wesley Brown, MD, Mentor, OH

Gastroenterologist: "Gutsy plot, not for the lily-livered."

Ivan Safonoff, MD, NYC, NY

Obstetrician: "Conceivably probable. Production should run nine months."

Ellen S. Goodrich, MD, Milledgeville, GA

Urologist: "A hesitant start; suspense builds URGENTLY with FREQUENCY of plot twist to a BURNING CLIMAX. I'd give it a three-glass rating."

John E. Glennon, MD, Granville, NY

Allergist: "Before last night, I would have scratched this season. This show is a real shot in the arm."

L. Robert Rubin, MD, Danbury, CT

COLLECTIVE NOUNS

ASSIGNMENT:
Ascribe names to grouped physicians, in the same vein as "a pride of lions, a bevy of beauties, a school of fish, a rafter (yes!) of turkeys."

EXAMPLES:
A brace of orthopedists
A murmuration of cardiologists
A smear of microbiologists

ENTRIES:
A Who's WHO of epidemiologists

> Dean A. Watson, MD, Midland, TX

A pleurality of pulmonologists

> Melvin J. Breite, MD, Bayside, NY

A detachment of retinal surgeons

> Jonathan S. Ehrlich, MD, Atlanta, GA

A tumescence of sex therapists

> Patrick M. Boccagno, MD, Altoona, PA

A crockful of psychiatrists

> James Mannion, MD, Redding, CA

An infantry of neonatologists

> James K. Sullivan, MD, Providence, RI

A crypt of deceased proctologists

> William V. Adler, MD, Downey, CA

A glomeration of nephrologists

> Sherri Chatham, LPN, Great Falls, MT

A floc of serologists

Louis Parham, MD, Hampton, VA

An invasion of cardiologists

Howard T. Chatterton, MD, Ladysmith, WI

A significant number of biostatisticians.

Doris E. Fletcher, Kendall park, NJ

A helix of geneticists

M. E. Carlin, MD, Miami, FL

ACRIMONIA

ASSIGNMENT:

Contrive a medical curse for some deserving offender.

EXAMPLES:

Seven exanthems upon you!

May the Joint Commission inflict grave doubts upon your hospital.

May you be plagued by nasal discharge and generalized pruritus when fully scrubbed, gowned, and gloved.

ENTRIES:

Please remember that you have Alzheimer's.

Edward M. Thompson, MD, Riverside, CA

May a morbidly obese patient mistake you for a gurney.

Marc Williams, MD, Riverside, CA

May you be some intern's "Great Case."

Robert J. Darios, MD, Lansing, MI

May your emergency calls coincide with the height of your lovemaking.

Dr. and Mrs. Grafton Fanney, Jr., Euclid, OH

And may the pot of gold at the end of your colonoscope turn into what usually is at the end of a colonoscope.

Melvin J. Breite, MD, Bayside, NY

May a blowfish attach to your indwelling catheter.

J. E. Mielcarek, DO, Las Vegas, NV

Peyronie's be damned! A double helix on your member!

Hugh H. Wang, MD, Clayton, CA

May your cremaster go into permanent tetany.

Richard A. Mingione, MD, Atlantic City, NJ

May the plaintiff discover your Swiss bank account.

Steven K. Bidleman, Klamath Falls, OR

May your severe benign ideopathic tinnitus commence with the downstroke of the baton on next opening night.

W. L. Mahon, Jr., MD, Carmichael, CA

May Schistosoma japonicum contaminate your Toyota.

M. Sharifi, MD, Waukegan, IL

May the tongues of one thousand grandmothers tell you how to treat your pediatric patients.

J. Patrick Evans, MD, Savannah, GA

SPECIALTY OF THE HOUSE

ASSIGNMENT:
Name a physician-owned restaurant appropriately.

EXAMPLES:
Neurologist—The Scrambled EEG
Pathologist—The Slide Inn
Chest surgeon—The Rib Cage

ENTRIES:
Gynecologist—Chlamydia Jane's Chlams and Crabs
> R. C. Whitesitt, MD, Helena, MT

Urologist—Turgor King
> Michael Ichniowski, MD, Lutherville, MD

Geriatrics—Al Zimer's Incontinental Cuisine
> Paul D. Ross, MD, Great Neck, NY

Pulmonologist—Hack's Open Air Spit
> Robert L. Hillery, MD, Findlay, OH

Gastroenterologist—High Fibes
> Renee Katz, Bronx, NY

Allergist—The Wheeze 'n' Eos Inn
> Henry J. Dold, MD, Arlington Heights, IL

Urologist—The Twisted Orchid Oyster House
> Eugene W. Arellano, MD, Glendale, CA

Microbiologist—Petri's Delicious Dishes
> Allan R. La Reau, MD, Kalamazoo, MI

Psychiatrist—The Oral Fixation
> Tabby Stone, MD, Studio City, CA

Neurologist—Guillain's Barre & Grille

Jonathan S. Ehrlich, MD, Atlanta, Georgia

Radiologist—Ray's Waffle House

Edward M. McMahon, Jr., MD, Seattle, WA

Rheumatologist/Orthopedist—The Joint Joint

Susan Lynn Ehlers, M.A., Seattle, WA

Proctologist—The Back Door

Doris Fletcher, Kendall Park, NJ

CINEMASCOPE

ASSIGNMENT:
Choose the title of any movie and give it a medical scenario.

EXAMPLES:
Hush . . . Hush, Sweet Charlotte: Deciding that silence is golden, terrorists attempt to extort ransom by deploying a laryngitis ray on a North Carolina city.

Rocky IV: With stones in each kidney, the gallbladder, and salivary duct, a patient's placement into the new quadritripter initiates events that build to a shattering climax.

Some Like It Hot: Genetically altered organisms thrive in an autoclave and emerge to invade. Ice bag barricades and an intrepid cryosurgical counterattack make for high drama.

ENTRIES:
The Seven Year Itch: Pruritic plague paralyzes Pittsburgh. Dust distributed by demonic dermatologist defies detectives. (Rated G—not a skin flick.)

Morey Filler, MD, San Francisco, CA

The Sterile Cuckoo: After vasectomy reversal fails, a deranged patient escapes from a mental institution and preys upon the nation's urologists, vowing that they all will share the same terrible fate.

Adrian J. Morris, MD, Dickson City, PA

High Noon: Brilliant ensemble cast dramatizes the true-life tribulations of a psychiatrist and his midday substance-abuse group.

Marc S. Williams, MD, Riverside, CA

Patton: The general survives the war to become a hospital administrator.

Joseph J. Richardson, MD, Rochester, NY

Hair: Knowing that Americans spend millions to remove body hair, money-hungry scientist adds a hirsutism-inducing agent to the water supply so that people must buy his depilatories.

Laura A. B. Cifelli, Flemington, NJ

The Thin Man: Psychotic anorexic scientist, angered by his doctors' efforts to cure his obsession, develops lipogenic agents, causing them to develop morbid obesity.

Grafton C. Fanney, MD, Euclid, OH

No Way Out: The gripping inside story of a young victim of esophageal stenosis and anal atresia.

Robert R. Jones, MD, Nevada, MO

On the Waterfront: The adventures of a young urology resident during a two-month rotation at the Incontinence Clinic.

Thuan L. Tran, MD, Claremont, CA

THE H.S. BEFORE RXMAS

ASSIGNMENT:
  Add a medical second line to any line from Clement Moore's
  "A Visit from St. Nicholas."

EXAMPLES:
  And mamma in her kerchief, and I in my cap,
  Were bless'd with a fav'rable anion gap.

  The stockings were hung by the chimney with care,
  Leaving double the count of malleoli bare.

  He spoke not a word but went straight to his work,
  Testing ankle and knee and bicipital jerk.

  But I heard him exclaim as he drove out of sight,
  "Happy Christmas to all, and to all a REM night!"

ENTRIES:
  A wink of his eye and a twist of his head—
  St. Nick and St. Vitus together in bed!
                    Meyer B. Hodes, MD, Oceanside, NY

  With a little old driver, so lively and quick—
  I knew in a moment his thyroid was sick.
                    Carlyn M. Kline, MD, St. Joseph, MO

  He had a broad face and a little round belly
  Due to genes and not steroids, with help from the deli.
                    Grafton C. Fanney, MD, Euclid, OH

  The stockings were hung by the chimney with care,
  In hopes that the Medicare checks would be there.
                    Charles W. Webb, MD, Owosso, MI

When out on the lawn there arose such a clatter,
Due to eight tiny reindeer with ol' Osgood-Schlatter.

Richard H. Morris, MD, Harrison, OH

When what to my wondering eyes should appear,
Bright swirls and light flashes, a migraine was near.

Russell J. Cox, MD, Gastonia, NC

With a little old driver, so lively and quick,
Despite being bit by the Lyme disease tick.

Joseph F. J. Curi, MD, Torrington, CT

'Twas the night before Christmas, when all through the house,
The beeper was beeping, arousing the spouse.

Ken T. Johnson, Jr., MD, Pineville, LA

HISTORY TAKING

ASSIGNMENT:

Alter the name of a historical personage to reflect a medical endeavor of a whimsical sort.

EXAMPLES:

Julius Seizure—Roman neurological pioneer

Pontius Palate—Patron saint of oral surgeons

Pauncho Villi—The first to point out the consequences of hyperabsorption

ENTRIES:

Thrombus Valva Medison—American inventor and anticoagulationist

Gary Davis, MD, Evanston, IL

Useless Grant—Government researcher

Gene Westveer, MD, Jenison, MI

Ortho von Birthmark—German dermatologist dealing in right-sided lesions.

Ronald L. Goldman, MD, San Francisco, CA

Errant Burr—First neurosurgeon to be sued for operating on the wrong side

Don N. Orelup, MD, Albia, IA

Pons de Leon—Eternally youthful neuroanatomist

Ted McMahon, MD, Seattle, WA

Toothloose Lautrec—Dental surgeon in a trauma center

Kenneth A. Deitcher, MD, Albany, NY

Louis Pasteurine—The first successful prostatectomy patient

Robert A. Fink, MD, Norfolk, VA

Mata Harakiri—German spy who underwent laparotomy for hiding secrets

Julio Novoa, MD, Lutherville, MD

Yohimbine Sebastian Bach—Upright organist/composer

Jerome J. Schneyer, Southfield, MI

Semen Bolivar—South America's Father of Artificial Insemination

Michael Hanson, MD, Fort Thomas, KY

Sir Alexander Phlegming—Nobel Prize winner for describing postnasal drip

R. M. Kniseley, MD, Boise, ID

Cathurine the Great—Urologists' patron saint

Grafton Fanney, MD, Euclid, OH

Marc Atony—Designer of the external uterine contraction monitor

David R. Fall, MD, Gillette, WY

BENEDICTA

ASSIGNMENT:
Bestow a good wish or blessing in medicalese.

EXAMPLES:
May your BUN not exceed your IQ.
May Babinski never attach his name to your plantar reflex.
May he remain invisible to PRO.

ENTRIES:
May the islets of Langerhans allow you to enjoy la dolce vita.

Joseph F. J. Curi, MD, Torrington, CT

May her streptococcal infection be quelled before St. Vitus's name appears on her dance card.

Donald Barkan, MD, Swampscott, MA

May the voices you hear always be of someone there.

Bob Darios, Lansing, MI

May your beeper go off as the committee meeting drags on.

A. R. La Reau, MD, Kalamazoo, MI

May your HMO have a 1% administrative cost and a 99% fee payment.

Joseph D. Richardson, MD, Rochester, IN

May you never suffer from a depilitating disease.

Renee Katz, Bronx, NY

May SOB in your chart be there for your attitude and not for an MI.

Julio Novoa, MD, Towson, MD

May your income double the amount you pay for malpractice insurance.

Robert L. Hillery, MD, Findlay, OH

May you be as good a doctor as your patients think you are.

Richard H. Morris, MD, Harrison, OH

May all of your drips be no worse than postnasal and all of your discharges from the National Guard.

Ray B. Vaughters, Jr., MD, Aiken, SC

May all your valves, channels, and orifices remain patent.

Meyer B. Hodes, MD, Oceanside, NY

May your breathalyzer numbers always fall below your bilirubin.

Eugene W. Arellano, MD, Glendale, CA

TOWERING BABEL

ASSIGNMENT:
Intone something medical in biblical terminology.

EXAMPLES:
And the Surgeon who is called General spake thusly: Ignite ye not the leaf of the tobacco lest it be thine own fiery furnace.

Yea, though I walk through the valley of cotton pledgets, I shall fear no weevil.

Spake the Chief of Service: For this plague of boils, let there be a staph conference to which all cometh.

ENTRIES:
Thus spake the prophet: When thou visitest the Land of Montezuma, drink not of the water, lest there come over thee the desolation of the Step which is called Quick.

Charles W. Webb, MD, Owosso, MI

Inasmuch as thou hast failed to follow thy diet, therefore, also, shall thy garments prove insufficient to cover thee.

Robert C. Whitesitt, MD, Helena, MT

Hark! Rise up, my beloved! For, lo, my follicles have ripened, the petri dishes are put forth; the time of ovulation is come, and the voice of the fertile is heard in our land.

Meyer B. Hodes, MD, Oceanside, NY

He that trusteth in his own heart is a fool, but he who so walketh to a second opinion, he shall be delivered.

Evelyn L. Weissman, MD, Malone, NY

And it came to pass that God created man. But it was the Devil that gaveth man a prostate.

Gerard K. Nash, DO, Amarillo, TX

And lo, the Healers did cry out, saying, "A scourge hath beset the land, causing the righteous to be afraid and the pure of heart to lament their fate."

But no one heeded their cries, and the plague soon beset the other inhabitants of the land. Who then bemoaned their plight: "Not fair; we thought only the healers to be afflicted and thus our hearts were closed to their pleas."

So the plague waxed stronger, and its forces, which were called HCFA, PRO, and MEDICARE, did scorn the people of the land, and proclaim: "Thus doth the politics of expediency bring forth its toll."

And the people turned once more to the Healers, saying: "Now we hath understanding. Help us again in the custom and manner of old." But the Healers were gone, and only the Bureaucrats were left to hear.

Mary E. Raum, MD, Ocala, FL

Goliath down, thou hast chronic fatigue.

Renee Katz, Bronx, NY

SIMILES

ASSIGNMENT:
Give instances of iatrotalk applied to as . . . as . . . situations.

EXAMPLES:
Mean as a PRO reviewer with Peyronie's and a traffic ticket.
Busy as a patient receiving diuretics, cathartics, and ipecac.
Unlikely as an office month without a dues notice, insurance premium, or donation solicitation.

ENTRIES:
Thin as the line between my Quality Medical Care and your Greedy Overutilization.

Don N. Orelup, MD, Albia, IA

As humiliating as missing the obvious.

Hugh H. Wang, MD, Clayton, CA

As wide as the emotional swing when the summons turns out to be for the reading of a lost relative's will.

Grafton C. Fanney, MD, Euclid, OH

Cacophonous as the obstetrician's phone ringing at 3:00 AM.

Morey Filler, MD, San Francisco, CA

Reliable as a color-blind laryngitic describing her rash over the telephone.

Robert L. Hillery, MD, Findlay, OH

Shaky as a patient with Graves' disease and rigor, who accidentally sat on a vibrator.

William V. Adler, MD, Downey, CA

Fragrant as an anaerobe.

Bernadine Z. Paulshock, MD, Wilmington, DE

As late as the day the rabbit died.

Paul C. Dolan, MD, Great Falls, MT

As numerous as unsolicited medical questions on your day off.

Russell J. Cox, MD, Gastonia, NC

Frantic as a hyperthyroid chihuahua in heat.

Edward M. Thompson, MD, Granite Falls, NC

Hyperkinetic as a "speed freak" with tinea cruris and Enterobius vermicularis infestation.

Joseph F. J. Curi, MD, Torrington, CT

FOREIGN BODIES

ASSIGNMENT:
Doctor any foreign word or expression to produce a medical meaning.

EXAMPLES:
Habeas carpus—The wrist surgery patient is ready.
Comme cecum ça—With this colonoscope I thee examine.
Charoscuro—¼ degree burn.
Feliz Ano Nuevo—Happy colostomy.

ENTRIES:
Casus belli—It's something you ate.
De gustibus non est disputandum—Yes, it's definitely something you ate.

> Ellen Conford, Great Neck, NY

In vena veritas—I'm really in the vein.

> Melvin J. Breite, MD, Bayside, NY

Honey soit qui mal y pons—Beware of sweets stuck in your brain.

> Morris Spielberg, MD, Brooklyn, NY

Gnome de plume—Autosomal recessive dwarf with long feathery hair.

> Alan Goldman, MD, Raleigh, NC

Expost fracto—If you run into the goalpost, you must expect to break something.

> Paul M. Dichter, MD, Massillon, OH

Esprit de corpse—Fun in the pathology department.

> Allen M. Perelson, MD, Buckingham, PA

Mi case es su case—Request for consultation.

> Mary E. Raum, MD, Ocala, FL

De gustibus non dispudenda—There's no accounting for gynecology.

Gary J. Davis, MD, Evanston, IL

Nicht wahr—Where did he cut himself?

Carlyn M. Kline, MD, St. Joseph, MO

Sick transit pyloria mundi—All enemas are fleeting.

Marc S. Williams, MD, La Crosse, WI

Zuppa ministone—A product of lithotripsy.

Melvin J. Breite, MD, Bayside, NY

Charcot à son gout—Oh, my swollen joints!

Doris E. Fletcher, Kendall Park, NJ

SPORTS MEDICINE

ASSIGNMENT:
Create athletic medical team names with a short explanation as to the appropriateness of such names.

EXAMPLES:
The Sclerae—Players noted for toughness and durability.
The Agglutinins—Masters of the team effort. Know how to stick together.
The Lithotripters—Crushingly hard-hitters.

ENTRIES:
Heimlichs (they never choke under pressure),
Doug Cook, MD, Ketchikan, AK

The Cryptorchites—Whiz kids famous for their hidden ball trick.
Joseph F. J. Curi, MD, Torrington, CT

The Hypodermics—Know how to stick it to 'em.
Robert W. Tufft, MD, Oakland, CA

The Lipodystrophies—Best wide ends in football
Joel T. Appleton, MD, Abilene, TX

The Gastric Acids—Always ready to steal a base.
Robert A. Fink, MD, Norfolk, VA

The Pituitaries—The sellar dwellers of the Cranial League.
Keith O. Wilson, MD, Ada, OK

The Villi—Able to absorb anything thrown at them.
Paul S. Sudack, MD, Miami Springs, FL

The Sphincters (nothing gets by them, and they have the best tight end in the business)?
Jonathan S. Ehrlich, MD, Atlanta, GA

The Maculae—Great vision shown in fielding a team . . . coned down to brightest performance . . . Coach Fovea says team focused . . . top contender for Optic Cup.

Marc S. Williams, MD, La Crosse, WI

. . . And a for-real softball team in Anderson, South Carolina, made up of family practice residents named the "Nads" . . . so the fans could yell, "Go *Nads*!"

Scott Counts, MD, Tulsa, OK

THE FIRING LINE

ASSIGNMENT:
How to express the state of dismissal of a health care worker?

EXAMPLES:
Gynecologist—Excolpated   Dentist—Uprooted

Cardiologist—Disheartened   Dermatologist—Downscaled

ENTRIES:
Gynecologist—XXed

Morey Filler, MD, San Francisco, CA

Microbiologist—Put out to Pasteur

H. Wesley Brown, MD, Mentor, OH

Thoracic surgeon—Redshirted

William O. Ameen, Jr., MD, Greensboro, NC

Neurologist—Uprooted

Kenneth R. Kellner, MD, Gainesville, FL

Bulemia specialist—Given the heave-ho

Lee S. Yosewitz, MD, Phoenix, AZ

Orthopedic technician—Outcast

Terry A. Hollenbeck, MD, Los Gatos, CA

Proctologist—Upended

Mark D. Stabler, MD, Deerfield Beach, FL

Oncologist—G-Phased out

Elms L. Allen, MD, Winston-Salem, NC

Nephrologist—Shut down

Grita Daum, MD, New York, NY

Otolaryngologist—Sent packing

Michael Ichniowski, MD, Lutherville, MD

Gastroenterologist—Dumped

Irving Thorne, MD, Minneapolis, MN

Fluid/electrolyte specialist—Debased

Alan Goldman, MD, Raleigh, NC

Infectious disease specialist—Victim of staph reduction

Carlyn M. Kline, MD, St. Joseph, MO

Dermatologist—Bumped [or scratched—Ed.]

Janet Johns, MD, Grand Rapids, MI

Surgeon—Cut back

Edward L. Zimney, MD, Wilmington, DE

IN SITU

ASSIGNMENT:
Select a location whose name would seem a natural habitat for some medical endeavor.

EXAMPLES:
Great Neck—Goiter treatment center
Bora Bora—Trephine and endoscopic works
El Salvador—Skin ointment manufacture

ENTRIES:
Appleton, WI—Municipality with no physicians
Jerome J. Schneyer, MD, Southfield, MI

Dripping Springs, TX—Center for enuresis alarm pads
Russell J. Cox, MD, Gastonia, NC

Patrickswell, Ireland—Center for study of peripheral edema in saints.
M. B. Hanson, MD, Fort Thomas, KY

Chartres—Medical records city
Anatoly Belilovsky, MD, Brooklyn, NY

Maldive Islands—Locale for swim team spine surgery
Mark Pashayan, MD, Gainesville, FL

Adelaide—Alzheimer's care center
Ralph French, MD, Anna Maria, FL

Lower Bucks County, PA—Where HMOs reign supreme
Sheila Gunning-Jass, Lawrenceville, NJ

South Bend—Center for descending colon surgery
H. Wesley Brown, MD, Mentor, OH

Malagasy Republic—Simethicone source
Charles G. Eschenburg, MD, Delray Beach, FL

Paw Paw (MI) and Walla Walla (WA)—Echolalia Treatment Centers, Inc.
Echolalia Treatment Centers, Inc.

Allan R. La Reau, MD, Kalamazoo, MI

Poconos—Nasal-packing material factory site

Michael Ichniowski, MD, Lutherville, MD

Yugoslavia—Center for hypersalivation treatment

Hugh H. Wang, MD, Clayton, CA

LETTERPERSONS

ASSIGNMENT:
Create a relative acronym for a medical organization.

EXAMPLES:
CORNEA: Convivial Ophthalmological Raconteurs Needing Eclectic Association

SCOPE: Society Composed of Penetrating Experts

MEATUS: Members Exemplary at Treating Urological Subjects

ENTRIES:
WHOOPS: World Hospital Organization of Operative Preventable Slipups

Hugh H. Wang, MD, Clayton, CA

FORCEPS: Federation of Resourceful Clinical Experts Preventing Sections

Julio Novoa, MD, Lutherville, MD

MQIMS (Pronounced "Mickey Mouse"): Medical Quality Inspection Management Systems

Don N. Orelup, MD, Albia, IA

PUMPITUP: Physicians' Union for Management and Promotion of Inflatable Transurethral Prostheses

Gary Davis, MD, Evanston, IL

STENT: Society to Expand Narrow Tunnels

Judy Reingold, MLS, Manchester, NH

!FEIRGDOOG: First Eclectic Insensible Ribald Gathering of Dyslexic Obstetricians, Orthodontists, and Geriatricians

Marvin G. Gregory, MD, Nashville, TN

GONAD: Genetic Overlay Nurturing Anatomical Duplication

Herbert Bandell, MD, Fontana, CA

RECTUM: Retentive Endoscopists Contemplating Their Ultimate Mission

Sherri Chatham, Great Falls, MT

TESTIS/TESTES: Transsexual Endocrine Society to Inhibit Spermatogenesis/ Traditional Endocrine Society to Enhance Spermatogenesis

Ivan Safonoff, MD, NYC, NY

LASER: Legendary Association Seeking Enlightened Retinologists

Stanley Hartness, MD, Kosciusko, MS

LIMITED PRACTICE

ASSIGNMENT:
In this era of specialization, contrive a super subsubspecialty.

EXAMPLES:
Levo-epistaxonomist—Bleeds of the sinistral nostril
Psychlist—Services peddled only to emotionally ill bikers
Seminole vesiculographer—Reproductive imaging of Native Americans

ENTRIES:
Cannesthesiologist—Sedatives to tension-ridden film festival nominees
J. Kirby Simon, New York, NY

Proctorlogist—Performance review of other specialists applying for hospital privileges
Anthony Somkin, MD, Berkeley, CA

Autolaryngologist—Fixes taxi drivers' vocal cords
Mark Pashayan, MD, Gainesville, FL

Sinistropolydactylectomizer—Removes supernumerary digits of left hand.
Edmund W. Kline, MD, St. Joseph, MO

Rectorectocorrectologist—Diseases of right side of distal colon
Melvin J. Breite, MD, Bayside, NY

Obstinatrician—Delivery services for only the tenaciously unyielding and pigheaded
Michael McNamara, MD, High Point, NC

Pheozuckerkandlologist—Pheochromocytomas of the Organ of Zuckerkandl
Paul J. Nuccio, MD, Tacoma, WA

Beadiatrician—Removal of foreign bodies from children's ears and noses

Michael Ichniowski, MD, Lutherville, MD

Amenorrheologist—Helping clergy fix (amend) overlong sermons

D. R. Downs, MD, Dodgeville, WI

Pedipodipediculopathist—Lice infestations of children's feet

Russell J. Cox, MD, Gastonia, NC

SLOGAN'S HEROES

ASSIGNMENT:
Attach a slogan or motto appropriate to the stationery and cards of a particular type of practice.

EXAMPLES:
Pulmonologist: "None shall disputum."
Vasectomist: "Emission impossible"
Fluid, electrolyte physiologist: "Follow the liter."
Hematologist: "Hematocritters"

ENTRIES:
Southwestern Medical oncologist: "Chemo Savvy"

Gary J. Coomber, MD, Santa Rosa, CA

Plastic surgeon: "A Stitch in Time Saves Thine."

Ralph French, MD, Anna Maria, FL

Psychiatrist: "I Shrink, Therefore, I Am."

Ivan F. Safonoff, MD, New York, NY

Obstetrician: "We Part Your Waters."

Allen M. Perelson, MD, Buckingham, PA

Sleep therapist: "Zzze Bezzzt."

Charles W. Webb, MD, Owosso, MI

Medical administrator: "Carpe Per Diem."

Ann E. Morrissey, MD, Chico, CA

Proctologist: "Best analyzers in town"

Michelle Perez, Coral Gables, FL

Radiologist: "X-Rated Professional"

Eric Diamond, MD, New York, NY

Epidemiologist: "If It's Contagious, We'll Catch It."

Edward M. Thompson, MD, Granite Falls, NC

Dermatologist: "Makes Derma Firma"

Mary E. H. Stark, Dalmatia, PA

MD expert witness: "Have Gun, Will Travel."

B. J. Cochrane, MD, Watertown, WI

Pacemaker cardiologist: "For the Times of Your Life"

Mark Pashayan, MD, Gainesville, FL

MRI radiologist: "It's the Next Best Thing to Being There."

Joseph B. Szgalsky, MD, Woodbury, NJ

YE OLDE PUTDOWNE

ASSIGNMENT:

Deprecate another's mentality with a verbal medical missile.

EXAMPLES:

A few islands short of a pancreas.
Never has more than one synapse firing at one time.
His/her glomeruli are open, but there's no filtration.

ENTRIES:

The oxygen's flowing, but there's no one inhaling.

Hugh H. Wang, MD, Clayton, CA

. . . standing in the shallow end of the gene pool.

Joseph F. Benenate, DO, Dallas, TX

. . . cervical vertebrae aren't weight-bearing.

Gary J. Davis, MD, Evanston, IL

Circle of Willis only reaches 350 degrees.

Donald Barkan, MD, Swampscott, MA

Organ donor material . . . ammonia level of Mr. Clean.

Anonymous Dr. S, Missouri

Lytes are on, but nobody's home.

M. David Lauter, MD, York, ME

4,256 genes . . . all recessive.

Robert H. Wilbee, MD, Las Cruces, NM

No traffic in his/her block; main artery completely closed.

Dr. and Mrs. Richard J. Stark, Herndon, PA

Always one sheet short and one bedpan behind.

Raymond Bechtle, Minnetonka, MN

. . . a walking argument against home deliveries.

James S. Bruce, MD, Milwaukee, WI

Why not upgrade to catatonia?

Ralph French, MD, Anna Maria, CA

Rolando vs. Silvius border dispute never settled.

Julio Novoa, MD, Lutherville, MD

Betz cell receptors only for testosterone.

Dr. Grafton Fanney, Jr., Euclid, OH

Eyes open but no potential evoked.

James A. Gamache, MD, Storm Lake, IA

A few disks shy of a full neck.

Wendy Moore, MA; Larry Maccree; and
Jeffrey Pearson, DO, San Marcos, CA

TO GIVE THANKS

ASSIGNMENT:
Express gratitude for some medical happening or non-happening.

EXAMPLES:
Because of a double X-ray error, I operated on the correct kidney.
I was called from the seminar just before the slide presentation (and how thankful I am that I thought to arrange it).
It wasn't blood after all—the gag involved Pyridium.

ENTRIES:
The successful Heimlich maneuver on my inebriated brother-in-law completely ruined his powder blue polyester leisure suit.

Joseph F. J. Curi, MD, Torrington, CT

He told me he was not sad with the diagnosis of Alzheimer's, in that he would have the chance to meet "knew" friends every day.

Julio Novoa, MD, Towson, MD

I forgot which twin I had diagnosed with EB viral infection, but it didn't matter . . . they were monozygotic.

Marc S. Williams, MD, La Crosse, WI

I mixed up the urines for the Friedman test, but since I used a male rabbit, it didn't make any difference.

Dr. Grafton C. Fanney, MD, Euclid, OH

The odor in the exam room was not from a dirty diaper after all, but only Limburger cheese being consumed by Mom.

Russell J. Cox, MD, Gastonia, NC

An ingrowing toenail impeded a promising career in ballet but produced an upstanding podiatrist.

Marvin G. Gregory, MD, Nashville, TN

A crash cart's head-on collision with a gurney on the way to pathology revived my hypothermic DOA.

Michael Anteski, MD, Brockton, MA

Fortunately I sustained a skull fracture: otherwise, my auto insurance would not have covered the broken windshield that my head went through.

Eugene W. Arellano, MD, Glendale, CA

I was greatly relieved as I awoke from my nap under the tree to find that the intermittently sharp, stabbing pain I felt in my forehead was caused only by a foraging woodpecker.

Melvin J. Breite, MD, Bayside, NY

Because of my known bilateral ptosis, no one can tell if I fall asleep at seminars.

Jeffrey Pearson, DO, San Marcos, CA

DECEMBER DESIDERATA

ASSIGNMENT:

What, medically, would you like for Christmas? State a preference.

EXAMPLES:

A self-irrigating catheter

A PRO freebie coupon book (each nullifying a censure)

A "smart" IV needle that never misses the vein

One-piece zip-up street clothes and ditto OR suit

ENTRIES:

Neonatal packets containing (1) one dozen self-cleaning diapers; (2) two nursing bottles that disintegrate after one year's use; and (3) one jar of spinach-flavored thumb dressing.

Robert R. Jones, MD, Nevada, MO

A labor-length regulator to time deliveries to coincide with committee meetings but that would avoid concerts, kids' ball games, anniversaries, and so on.

David C. Swanson, MD, Marshall, MN

An Alzheimer variant afflicting only tort lawyers of all ages.

C. A. Somaskanda, MD, Sodus, NY

A pediatric tongue blade that does not induce the familiar gag reflex that ruins my favorite ties.

Joseph F. J. Curi, MD, Torrington, CT

A robot that can read my mind and knows which mails should be trashed without being opened.

Cosme R. Cagas, MD, Belleville, IL

Remote-control bedpans with automatic turbo-powered wash.

Sherri Chatham, LPN, Great Falls, MT

A drug that quickly and safely dissolves adipose tissue.

Doris Fletcher, Kendall Park, NJ

A beeper that goes off for only really important calls.

L. Scott Herman, MD, San Gabriel, CA

A fetal alarm clock (labor preset for 7:00 AM).

Morey Filler, MD, San Francisco, CA

A computerized finger insert that records the correct diagnosis.

Robert Pearson, DO, Emerson, NJ

A pair of MRI-specs to replace now-outdated X-ray specs.

Jeffrey Pearson, DO, San Marcos, CA

Wide-angle glasses to enable my specialist colleagues to see the whole patient.

Dr. Grafton C. Fanney, Jr., Euclid, OH

A computerized medical answering machine that doles out the correct medical advice to all who phone after 11:00 PM on on-call nights.

Russell J. Cox, MD, Gastonia, NC

ALLITERATIONAL

ASSIGNMENT:
Contrive medical phraseology with a repetitive first letter.

EXAMPLES:
Industrious islets of insulinism
Compensation-cropping committees cutting care costs callously
Subscapular sign of stone-spasm syndrome

ENTRIES:
The psad and psorry pspectacle of psoft, psatiny pskin pscarred and pscaled with psoriasis

Gary Davis, MD, Evanston, IL

Timely telltale Tzanck test thwarts theoretically troublesome titillating tryst.

Joseph F. J. Curi, MD, Torrington, CT

Treating PMS: Overcoming occasional overbearing ovarian occurrences

Joseph M. Eder, MD, West Hills, CA

The malignant mandible manufactures more malicious mischief than man can manage.

Perry S. MacNeal, MD, Moorestown, NJ

Optic opportunist opted for ophthalmology over optometry for overtly obvious opulence.

Irving Thorne, MD, Minneapolis, MN

Persnickety pagers pose penchant pertaining to persistent peskiness precisely at pinnacle of passion.

Hugh H. Wang, MD, Clayton, CA

The particular painful pressing pressure problem of prostatitis

Michael J. Zappitelli, DO, Norristown, PA

Cardiologists caution: Cut cholesterol, count calories, keep coronaries clear.

Doris E. Fletcher, Kendall Park, NJ

Perenially peripatetic paradox perpetually pursues postgraduate pearls, purportedly perfecting professional prescriptive patterns.

Drs. Edmund and Carlyn Kline, St. Joseph, MO

Fecund females feeling fetuses frolicking freely in fundic fluidity

Charles W. Webb, MD, Owosso, MI

Instant infant: Fat, fecund Fanny's fifth fetus fell from Fanny fleetly, face first, floorward, forcing flutters for four frozenly fixed, frustrated phobic physicians, fearing fetal failure and favoring forceps.

Melvin J. Breite, MD, Bayside, NY

LOVERLY

ASSIGNMENT:
For Valentine's Day, think of something that doctors love.

EXAMPLES:
Colleagues who dial the phone themselves

Benevolent JCAH examiners

Nearby inexpensive CME courses yielding many credit hours and useful information

Pharmacists who answer the phone themselves

ENTRIES:
. . . to be chosen for a second opinion for lateral chest wall pain on the day the herpetic vesicles appear

> C. N. Young, MD, Loves Park, IL

. . . patients who don't keep their insurance checks

> J. G. Porterfield, MD, Memphis, TN

. . . parents who do not threaten their children with a shot from the doctor

> Carlyn M. Kline, MD, St. Joseph, MO

. . . attorneys (a comic valentine)

> Morey Filler, MD, San Francisco, CA

. . . bacteria that cooperate with the antibiotic

> Ralph French, MD, Anna Maria, FL

. . . that the most argumentative doctor on the staff will forget to attend the monthly meeting

> Dr. Michael J. Zappitelli, Norristown, PA

. . . those hospital switchboards with real live operators

> Paul S. Sudack, MD, Miami Springs, FL

. . . patients who do not have relatives practicing at the Mayo Clinic

Thuan L. Tran, MD, Claremont, CA

. . . an insurance agent who says, "You really have all you'll ever need."

Robert C. Whitesitt, MD, Helena, MT

. . . the last appointment of the day canceled by patient with somatization disorder, replaced by kid with healed cut needing slip for school, new Band-Aid, and no conversation.

Don N. Orelup, MD, Albia, IA

. . . mothers who take the soiled diapers with them instead of sneaking them into the exam room trash can.

Alan L. Goldman, MD, Raleigh, NC

. . . understandable journal articles that are applicable to clinical practice.

Russell J. Cox, MD, Gastonia, NC

THE EMERALD GUILE

ASSIGNMENT:
A well-intentioned but hard-of-hearing leprechaun mishears a request and grants a wish, with unexpected consequences.

EXAMPLES:
I asked for the touch of Midas and got a touch of epididymitis.
Help with taxes . . . epistaxis.
A cash start . . . a crash cart
Mental distractions . . . dental extractions
Of filial bond, a whit . . . an ileal conduit
A cure for myasthenia . . . curare for myasthenia

ENTRIES:
Asked: Admission to the medical center.
Received: Audition with the meddlesome censor.

> Hugh H. Wang, MD, Clayton, CA

Asked: Many years. Received: Ménière's.

> Sylvia Bernstein, Far Rockaway, NY

An X-ray report . . . an X-rated retort

> Russell J. Cox, MD, Gastonia, NC

Pleasant attention . . . placental retention

> Julio Novoa, MD, Lutherville, MD

Pirouettes in Rome . . . Tourette's syndrome

> Nita Coleman, MD, Elizabeth City, NC

A bottle in front of me . . . A frontal lobotomy

> Sheridan Anderson, MD, Grand Island, NE
> Charles H. Ayers, MD, Hawaiian Gardens, CA

Stopping the Peyronie's . . . Topping with pepperoni

> Dr. A. Somaskanda, Sodus, NY

The peat moss of Erin . . . Weak loss of urine

Donald Barkan, MD, Swampscott, MA

Expensive cabinetry, TV . . . Extensive cavitary TB

Ivan M. Safonoff, MD, NYC, NY

A chest of gold . . . A chesty cold

Forrest P. White, MD, Norfolk, VA

A home with a Cadillac . . . Glaucoma with cataracts

Jeff and Sharon White, Louisville, CT

A fax from Elvis . . . A fractured pelvis

Samuel A. Brewton, Jr., MD, Thomaston, GA

Pair of tights . . . Parotitis

H. Wesley Brown, MD, Mentor, OH

RUSSIAN DRESSINGS

ASSIGNMENT:
Russianize anything concerning the health care industry.

EXAMPLES:
Uralolologist: Authority on the verumontanum

Leon Trotsky: Bolshevik physician who first advocated the benefits of jogging

Irkutsk: myringotomy

Grigory Rasputum: Noted mucomystic

ENTRIES:
Rimsky-Korsakov: Bronchitis peculiar to tire repairmen
> R. C Whitesitt, MD, Helena, MT

Bladdervastuck: Pelvic trauma as described by Siberian ER physician
> Russell J. Cox, MD, Gastonia, NC

Drs. Ob, Lena, and Yenesei, PA: North Asia's largest uralogic drainage group
> Charles G. Eschenburg, MD, Delray Beach, FL

Maxim Gorky: An admitting intern's worst nightmare
> Melvin J. Breite, MD, Bayside, NY

Boris Gudenov: The end result of most medical school lectures
> Marc S. Williams, MD, La Crosse, WI

Eucrania: Universal headache remedy
> Meyer B. Hodes, MD, East Rockaway, NY

Anton Cheekoff: Noted head and neck surgeon as well as director of the Cheery Orchard, a facility for depressed Russian aristocrats.
> Ivan M. Safonoff, MD, New York, NY

Caucasus Coccus Caucus: Georgian bacteriologists' convention.
> Gary J. Coomber, MD, Santa Rosa, CA

The Baltics: Microscopic agents causing scrotal Lyme

Robert M. Pickoff, MD, Somerset, NJ

Byelorussian: Aftermath of fatty meal ingestion

Michael B. Hanson, MD, Fort Thomas, KY

Peter the Grate: Physician noted by colleagues for obnoxious personality

Sam Brewton, MD, Thomaston, GA

Rubleola: Disease characterized by one hundred kopeck spots.

Donald Barkan, MD, Swampscott, MA

Sputnik: Small sputum sample

H. Wesley Brown, MD, San Francisco, CA

Comrade: Minidose of radiation therapy

Carlyn Kline, MD, St. Joseph, MO

SHORT BOOKS

ASSIGNMENT:
Provide a title to a book of the medical genre, sure to be on the thin side.

EXAMPLES:
Ways to a Satisfactory Sitz Bath
We Were Wrong: A Compendium of Malpractice Lawyers' Voluntary Admissions of Unjust Litigation
The Treatment of Blisters: A Symposium

ENTRIES:
The Marlboro Man's Guide to a Healthy Heart
> C. J. Li, MD, New York, NY

Radiologists' Guide to Compact Cars
> Ted McMahon, MD, Seattle, WA

The Wit of Hospital Administrators
> Jeffrey Preston Weitzner, MD, Jacksonville, FL

Great Tales of Humble Neurosurgeons
> Forrest P. White, MD, Norfolk, VA

Directory of Medical Specialists Available for Consultations after 5:00 PM Friday
> Michael Brown, MD, Seneca, SC

Dissertation on Proper Location and Insertion of an Enema Tip
> Herman E. Schaffer, MD, Abilene, TX

Skin Tags—The Early Years
> Jonathan S. Ehrlich, MD, Atlanta, GA

Skin Words: Monosyllabic Dermatologic Diagnoses
> H. Wesley Brown, MD, Mentor, OH

Patients Who Prefer to Follow Their Hairdressers' Medical Advice—
Exploring the Logic

Kathleen M. Sheehan, MD, Tacoma, WA

Symposium: On Giving Free Medical Care to the Palm Beach
Retirement Home for Malpractice Lawyers

Grafton C. Fanney, MD, Euclid, OH

A Teaching Hospital Reference Guide to Competent Local Medical
Doctors

Martin J. Sinaisky, MD, Van Nuys, CA

How to Come out Ahead on Your Malpractice Premiums

F. P. Ambrose, MD, Coeur d'Alene, ID

The DRG Guide to Long-Term Hospitalization

Doris E. Fletcher, Kendall Park, NJ

FEAR ITSELF

ASSIGNMENT:
Coin a name for a special type of dread (-*phobia*).

EXAMPLES:
Magnifrancodilatophobia—Fear of passage of large-caliber urethral sounds

Mulitprobodurostikkophobia—Fear of difficult lumbar punctures

Thereocompensomagnobukkophobia—Fear of excessive medical bills

Interrogatobeaurocraciphobia—Fear of PRO

ENTRIES:
Litigaligaphobia—Fear of lawsuit over a misplaced suture

James R. Eelkema, MD, Bloomington, MN

Prolapsoproctophobia—Fear of falling behind

Joseph Grayzel, MD, Englewood, NJ

Dg Ru Ur Gd ophobia—Fear of drug-drug interactions

David Cameron, MD, Cincinnati, OH

Felinicerebroclaustrophobia—Fear of CAT scans

Alan M. Perelson, MD, Buckingham, PA

Flatulophilharmonicophobia—Fear of colonic accident during quiet lull between symphonic movements of community concert

Robert R. Johns, MD, Springfield, VT

Megalodigitusgynecopelviphobia—Fear of gynecologists with large hands

M. Gary Robertson, MD, Grand Haven, MI

Fallowphallophobia—Fear of impotence

Irving Thorne, MD, Minneapolis, MN

Puncturaduohemophobia—Fear of being stuck twice for blood

David P. Frelinger, MD, El Segundo, CA

OOophobia—Fear of not being reimbursed for services

Morey Filler, MD, San Francisco, CA

Tardifiloformophobia—Fear of missing the deadline for filing insurance claim forms

Robert M. Pickoff, MD, Somerset, NJ

Julyoneophobia—Fear of new interns

Robert A. Fink, MD, Norfolk, VA

Nocturnaphoniapediacalculasalicyliphobia—Fear of that after-midnight wake-up call requesting a toddler's dosage of aspirin

Joseph F. J. Curi, MD, Torrington, CT

Mitteladminoformophobia—Fear of third-party paperwork

Hugh H. Wang, MD, Clayton, CA

DEAD GIVEAWAYS

ASSIGNMENT:

Transplant an MD into another line of work and show how the vernacular tips his/her hand.

EXAMPLES:

Sportscaster: "He takes a right to the maxilla, throws a left to the epigastrium.

Carpenter: "A direct and indirect cabinet repair was performed."

Butcher: "This is a low-adipose, high-LDL cut."

Bus driver: "Insert exact fare into the foramen."

Fish bait merchant: "Viable annelids."

ENTRIES:

Quarterback: "It will be a pseudo-dextro handoff and a levo rollout on III."

Russell J. Cox, MD, Gastonia, NC

Radio patrolman: "At the decussation of 42nd and Park, I've got a car in the left lateral decubitus position."

Wilmot S. McCullough, III, MD, Sumter, SC

Baseball umpire: "You're excised!"

Melvin J. Breite, MD, Bayside, NY

Carnival barker: "Step right up and hear the exogenously obese lady sing!"

Marvin G. Gregory, MD, Nashville, TN

Mattress inspector: "The turgor is not resilient on palpation!"

Morris Spielberg, MD, Brooklyn, NY

Car mechanic: "We rehydrated the cooling system, did a water pump transplant, debrided the air filter, disimpacted the fuel line, and removed a foreign body from the tailpipe."

Kenneth Hurwitz, MD, Park City, UT

Dam builder: "I shall convert that wildly incontinent stream into an electrifyingly insignificant trickle."

David J. Schwartz, MD, Vineland, NJ

Auto-racing sportscaster: "He's threading his way incisively and making rapid anterior progress."

Chester S. Suske, DO, Deerfield, MA

Stand-up comedian: "Take my 46XX phenotypically female mate—please!"

Jonathan S. Ehrlich, MD, Atlanta, GA

Economist: "The general malaise prevalent in the economy can be at least partially ameliorated by bold reductive surgery on the debilitatingly high interest rates.

A. Somaskanda, MD, Sodus, NY

Clockmaker: "Perfect time; sinus bradycardia at sixty ticks a minute."

Donald Barkan, MD, Swampscott, MA

THE SWISS CONNECTION

ASSIGNMENT:
Append a medical addition to the Swiss Army knife.

EXAMPLES:
Thermometer for those who describe symptoms at social gatherings
Magnifying glass for the superfine print of medicine package inserts
Cigarette snuffer for the general welfare

ENTRIES:
Mini TV to watch football at medical staff meetings

> Morey Filler, MD, San Francisco, CA

Magnifying glass for examining Medicare payments

> Bernadine Z. Paulshock, MD, Wilmington, DE

Fourteen-gauge needle (there is no body cavity that cannot be reached with a strong arm and a FGN)

> Marc S. Williams, MD, La Crosse, WI

Compliance indicator—*Did* the patient really take the medicine as directed?

> Russell J. Cox, MD, Gastonia, NC

Compass to direct emergency exit from staff meeting

> Lourdes Romano-Jana, MD, Erie, PA

Telescoping trocar for emergency drainages, reversing to antenna for wider beeper range

> Charles G. Eschenburg, MD, Delray Beach, FL

Hedge trimmer for reading typical radiology report

> Charles W. Webb, MD, Owosso, MI

Master key to open all IRS, hospital administration, PRO, and expert witness secret files.

> C. N. Young, MD, Rockford, IL

Collapsible retrospectoscope to avoid PRO-denied admissions
Henry L. Harrell, MD, Ocala, FL

Whistle for refereeing intrafamily arguments in the hall
Jeffrey N. Graves, MD, Norfolk, VA

Miniature shovel for the stories heard in the doctors' lounge
Alvin Shulklapper, MD, New Rochelle, NY

Syringe of sodium pentothal (truth serum) for use at the convention of the American Society of Professional Witnesses
F.P. Ambrose, MD, Coeur d'Alene, ID

Pair of scales for weighing Relative Values
Thomas J. Durkin, MD, Ft. Washington, PA

APPELLATION SPRING

ASSIGNMENT:
Create a medical person whose name is appropriate to his/her field of practice.

EXAMPLES:
Said Hertz, gallbladder surgeon
Mehta Tarsal, podiatrist
Sue Damonas, infectious diseases
Dee Livery, obstetrics
Ira Spire, pulmonologist

ENTRIES:
Billie D. Kidd, née Stone, nephrologist

Andrea J. Pederson and Roger Gray, Chicago, IL

César Ian Seccione, Latin obstetrician with Scottish mother

Janice Krakora-Looby, MD, Vernon Hills, IL

Perry and Neil Natal, high-risk obstetricians

Gary D. Blake, MD, San Diego, CA

P. Oliver Mey, pediatrician

Doris Fletcher, Kendall Park, NJ

Cal Q. Li, urologist

Eugene W. Arellano, MD, Glendale, CA

Guy Dwyer, vascular surgeon

Michael G. Marre, MD, Las Vegas, NV

Len Simplant, ophthalmologist

Frank Reynolds, MD, Mililani, HI

Jewell Anna Lyzer, female male-infertility specialist

Marvin G. Gregory, MD, Nashville, TN

Miss Alline Meant, aspiring chiropractor
> R. M. Pettit, MD, Rochester, MN

Seymour Abner Maladies, diagnostician
> Gary Davis, MD, Evanston, IL

Al E. O'Morph, geneticist
> Charles G. Eschenburg, MD, Delray Beach, FL

Ol' Pop Smear, retired gynecologist
> Robert M. Pickoff, MD, Somerset, NJ

Hugh Remia, nephrologist
> Karl Brandspigel, MD, Elizabeth City, SC

Dennis L. Boe, sports physician
> George A. Wahlert, Brooklyn, NY

UNINITIATION RITES

ASSIGNMENT:

Give instances as to the way medical words may be misinterpreted by nonmedical listeners.

EXAMPLES:

Cochlear—Pertaining to a soft drink

Hippocampus—A college rich in weightlifters, shot-putters, and footballers

GI series—A military baseball competition

ENTRIES:

Krebs cycle: The Schwinn competition

Ivan M. Safonoff, MD, New York, NY

Intussusception: What the cornerback did to the quarterback

Melvin J. Breite, MD, Bayside, NY

Calcium channel blocker: Limestone formation hazardous to shipping

Arnold A. Yap, Alpine, NJ

Left costal margin: California

Edward M. McMahon, MD, Seattle, WA

Countershock: Reaction to supermarket prices

Harry W. Eichenbaum, MD, St. Petersburg, FL

Redundant colon: : :

Doris E. Fletcher, Kendall Park, NJ

Benign: Occasionally the last word called before "Bingo"

Michael J. Kelly, MD, Buffalo, IA

Syndrome: Evangelistic amphitheater

Frederick Schaffner, MD, Thousand Oaks, CA

Scala vestibuli: Milanese opera anteroom

Meyer B. Hodes, MD, Oceanside, NY

"Alice." Kelly: To the awake surgical patient, the most popular nurses in every operating room.

Sonja Carroll, MD, Cincinnati, OH

Hydrocephalus: VD acquired while swimming

Virginia Shipman, MD, Bartlesville, OK

Endorphin: Youngest parentless child

Gerald L. Haas, DO, Albia, IA

Ureteric calculus: Advanced math course

A. Somaskanda, MD, Sodus, NY

Subarachnoid: Lower than spiders on the evolutionary scale

Alan L. Goldman, MD, Raleigh, NC

POLITICAL PARADOX

ASSIGNMENT:
Speak of a political opponent in innocent medical terms that sound anything but innocuous. Let the opponent be a doctor.

EXAMPLES:
MY OPPONENT . . .

Is guilty of left-axis deviation.
Is a card-carrying member of the ACS.
Is soft on botulism.
Does nothing about the pulse deficit.

ENTRIES:
. . . was institutionalized after a cardiac arrest by infarcting in an all-male gym.

Stephen L. Kaufman, MD, San Francisco, CA

. . . has trickle-down incontinence.

Donald E. Loew, MD, Attleboro, MA

. . . publicly osculated his pregnant wife, causing her to rubricate.

Patrick M. Boccagno, MD, Altoona, PA

. . . is a Hippocrate of the highest order.

Steve Hardy, DO, Erie, PA

. . . has sinusoidal tendencies.

Michelle Tauber, MD Hana, HI

. . . has colonoscoped hundereds of persons while their backs were turned.

Jeffrey Pearson, DO, San Marcos, CA

. . . is nonspecific on urethritis.

Douglas Cook MD, Ketchikan, AK

. . . is against the farm belt. He said that he abhors vegetative states

R. E. Drawdy, MD, Plant City, FL

. . . has fallen into the grippe of Asian influenza.

Edward M. Sessa, MD, Schenectady, NY

. . . supports decapitation of the HMO-insured.

Robert A. Fink, MD, Norfolk, VA

. . . was a resident in a state psychiatric institution for three years.

Carlyn M. Kline, MD, St. Joseph, MO

. . . is not a mental giant; there's a void in his micturition.

Joseph D. Robertson, MD, Crossville, TN

. . . Energy program? Even his antibodies are antinuclear!

Jonathan S. Ehrlich, MD, Atlanta, GA

. . . may be an MD, and a PhD but is BS in the first degree.

Marvin G. Gregory, MD, Nashville, TN

. . . has accepted declared indigents with no remuneration whatsoever!

Meyer B. Hodes, MD, Oceanside, NY

GUARANTEED TO HAPPEN

ASSIGNMENT:

Invent a statement to precede an event that is sure to follow.

EXAMPLES:

Catheterization for retention: "For that which we are about to receive . . ."

Icebag application: "This may be cold comfort."

Venipuncture for fluids: "Welcome to the IV League."

Electroshock therapy: "This may change your mind."

ENTRIES:

Amputation of a genius's leg: "I've always wanted to stump the experts."

E. D. Morton, MD, Ogden, UT

Proctoscopy: "Rejoice, for there is light at the end of the tunnel."

Bruce J. Cochrane, MD, Watertown, WI

Penile implant: "You may be a little stiff in the morning."

Linda J. Lemay, MD, Cazenovia, NY

Sigmoidoscopy: "This is a stickup."

David Taube, MD, Hana, HI

Audiology testing: "Now hear this! Now hear this!"

Joanne Iacovino, MD, Salem, OR

Catheterization for retention: "Aprés moi le dèluge."

Jonathan S. Ehrlich, MD, Atlanta, GA

Presenting the bill: "Ask not what your doctor can do for you . . ."

Ivan M. Safonoff, MD, New York, NY

Removal of silicone implant: "Let's make a clean breast of it."

Carlyn M. Kline, MD, St. Joseph, MO

Pediatrician about to remove a splinter: "Hi-yo sliver, away!"
> Alan Goldman, MD, Raleigh, NC

Bunionectomy: "[Now for] the agony of de feet."
> Burnell Stripling, MD, Marinette, WI

Cardioversion: "This may come as a shock to you!"
> Shashi K. Agarwal, MD, Orange, NJ

DC cardioversion: "You may get a slight charge out of this."
> Stephen J. Hardy, DO, Erie, PA

Intramuscular injection: "Finally you are getting the point."
> Robert Pearson, DO, Emerson, NJ

Plantar wart treatment: "These are the times that try men's soles."
> Hugh Wang, MD, Clayton, CA

IT'S THE LAW

ASSIGNMENT:

Inspired by Murphy's law, devise a medical one, replete with misfortune. You may attach your name to it alliteratively.

EXAMPLES:

Sitters are found for quiet children. Hyperactive ones come to the office.

When your time is at a strict premium, the anesthetist will have trouble getting the spinal in.

As the patient count increases, phone calls square and paperwork cubes.

ENTRIES:

Paulshock's principle: Blood prefers to be transfused into the wrong person.

Bernadine Z. Paulshock, MD, Wilmington, DE

Bux's belief: When the diagnostic endoscope enters the body, the bleeding stops.

Robert B. Bux, MD, London, KY

Curi's comment: Nine times out of ten, the patient who slips on the ice in your parking lot has a relative who is a lawyer.

Joseph F. J. Curi, MD, Torrington, CT

Toni's truism: If you are running late, there will be no no-show patients.

Toni Brayer, MD, San Francisco, CA

Payne's postulate: One gets 85% of his phone calls from 15% of the patients.

William Payne, MD, Jackson, MI

Thomas's theorem: No matter what the time, the buzzer will go off just as you are about to eat.

Corollary: The number of pages received is directly related to the number of hours since you last ate.

Karen A. Thomas, MD, Bath, NC

Capps's canon: The more urgent-looking the mail, the less important the contents.

John L. Capps, MD, Gastonia, NC

Hodes's hypothesis: Chest auscultation in the elderly induces logorrhea.

Meyer B. Hodes, MD, Oceanside, NY

Arnold's axiom: The amount of a child's fighting against a procedure is directly proportional to the number of times "It won't hurt" is told him/her.

Arnold S. Goldstein, MD, Highland Park, IL

Martin's musing: It is impossible for a labor patient to progress from 3 cm. to complete in fifteen minutes unless the attending physician is home in bed.

Martin J. Sinaisky, MD, Van Nuys, CA

Morey's maxim: The last patient of the day invariably has thirteen chief complaints, twelve other physicians, eleven medicines, ten drug allergies, and is late for the appointment.

Morey Filler, MD, San Francisco, CA

IT SPEAKS VOLUMES

ASSIGNMENT:
Let an inquiring patron come up against a hospital librarian who has an unhelpful answer to any inquiring doc's question.

EXAMPLES:
Q: Do you have any books on arrhythmias?
A: They're in the atrium.

Q: Do you have any books on psychometric testing?
A: Scores of them.

Q: Do you have a book on equilibrium?
A: It's in the vestibule.

ENTRIES:
Q: . . . allergies to mustard seeds?
A: But of course.*

Joseph F. J. Curi, MD, Torrington, CT

Q: . . . Alzheimer's?
A: Four o'clock.

Morey Filler, MD, San Francisco, CA

Q: . . . obesity?
A: In the rotunda.

Jonathan S. Ehrlich, MD, Atlanta, GA

Q: . . . pediatrics?
A: Yes. See the shelf. See the books. See the books on the shelf.

Sylvia Bernstein, Far Rockaway, NY

---

* Those who questioned this seemingly irrelevant response failed to recall a popular ad for Grey Poupon mustard, in which a verbal exchange occurred about the product between men in two Rolls Royces.

Q: . . . spinal surgery?
A: We did until we cut back.

David Cameron, MD, Cincinnati, OH

Q: . . . diseases of the tongue?
A: Yes, but they're rather tasteless.

W. E. Watkins, MD, Nampa, ID

Q: . . . stress testing?
A: Take the stairs to the 24th floor.

S. Bharath, MD, Devils Lake, ND

Q: . . . the vagus nerve?
A: Wander around and you'll find it.

Kay Heggestad, MD, Madison, WI

Q: . . . transurethral prostatectomy?
A: Reams of them.

Dewey R. Heetderks, MD, Grand Rapids, MI

Q: . . . the Genome Project?
A: Yes—up the spiral stairs.

Robert C. Hauck, MD, Seattle, WA

Q: . . . the bronchial tree?
A: Try one of our branches.

Marvin C. Gregory, MD, Nashville, TN

Q: . . . the definition of amenorrhea?
A: No. Period.

Sharon M. Wallace, DO, Pensacola, FL

Q: . . . on the carpal bones?
A: I have one on hand.

Hal C. Scherz, MD, San Diego, CA

Q: . . . ACE inhibitors?
A: Do an about f—, take three p—s, and you'll be in the right pl—and pe—be with you.

Melvin G. Breite, MD, Bayside, NY

CABINETRY

ASSIGNMENT:
Conceive medical cabinet posts exclusive of Surgeon General.

EXAMPLES:
Secretary of Labor: Administrator of all delivery rooms
The Purgeon General: Cathartics czar
Secretary of the Interior: Regulator of anatomy curricula

ENTRIES:
Secretary of Traffic and Transportation: Manager of root and ear canals, carpal tunnels, dental bridges, femoral bypasses, aortic outflows, afferent arteries, and neural pathways

Carlyn Kline, MD, St. Joseph, MO

Joint Sheaves of Chaff: Utilization Review comes to Washington

Edward M. Sessa, MD, Schenectady, NY

Treachery Secretary: Generic bait-and-switch processor

Jayant Malhotra, MD, Homewood, IL

Chairman, Chief of Joint Staffs: Head of panel of rheumatology experts

Joseph Bernstein, MD, Philadelphia, PA

Minister of Foreign Affairs: Pediatric endoscopist

Julio Novoa, MD, Lutherville, MD

Attorney Genital: Protector of sexual rights

Hugh H. Wang, MD, Clayton, CA

Surgeon Generous: Administrator of all willing to accept Medicaid

David A. Kline, MD, Los Angeles, CA

Joint Chiefs: National instructors on how not to inhale

Gene Westveer, MD, Zeeland, MI

Secretary of the Triagery: Administrator of national emergency services

Jonathan Kurland, MD, Orinda, CA

Maternity General: The mother of all generals

Mary C. Vetro, Cheshire, CT

Secretary of Health and Human Services: Arranger of Chinese takeout for committee meetings on health care reform

Jeffrey Pearson, DO, San Marcos, CA

Secretary of Deferens: Oversees a vas network of supply tubules

Glenn H. Perelson, MD, Bonita, CA

Secretary of the Treasury Chest: Chief of all augmentation mammoplasties

Marvin G. Gregory, MD, Nashville, TN

Attorney Generous: No one qualified for this cabinet post

Alan M. Wagner, MD, Milwaukee, WI

AFFINITIES

ASSIGNMENT:
Fashion a word, suffix *-philia*, that embodies some practice-related pleasure.

EXAMPLES:
Holocompensaphilia: Love of 100% reimbursement for the amount billed

Barristopratfallophilia: Enjoyment of damaging embarrassment to malpractice lawyers

Fillofullofilophilia: Joy in having a large volume of patient records

Enucleophilia: Pleasure in shelling things out

ENTRIES:
Nocturnapedi-amifortisobstetrirepudia-appetitivictuslegitilarumcontracesa-reprovaginumnataliaphilia: Admiration by on-call pediatrician who, after hours, ignores hunger concerns and malpractice fears and, instead of performing a convenient C-section, patiently awaits a natural delivery.

Joseph F. J. Curi, MD, Torrington, CT

Rectodynia-adiosophilia: Joy of "losing" a problem patient to another office

Floyd T. Nasuti, MD, Philadelphia, PA

Alterojudiciophilia: Love of tort reform

Irving Thorne, MD, Minnepolis, MN

Cuproustau-introphilia: Love of inserting Copper-T IUDs.

Neal Green, MD, Corsicana, TX

Absentiomaternoneuroticaphilia: Joy experienced when the child with the hyper mother is a no-show.

C. M. Cunningham, MD, Columbia, SC

Utiloyoutoolatenofeeyouphilia: Pleasure in denying reimbursement

Edward M. Sessa, MD, Schenectady, NY

Tearenfilenforgetophilia: Pleasurable sensation of ripping apart journals, filing relevant articles, and never looking at them again

Marc S. Williams, MD, La Crosse, WI

Primo-effecto-economicophilia: Joy of success with the first-used and cheapest drug

Grafton C. Fanney, Jr., MD, Euclid, OH

Nomocesariophilia: The happiness of giving up obstetrics

Morey Filler, MD, San Francisco, CA

Claustrophilia: Love of the MRI machine

Melvin J. Breite, MD, Bayside, NY

Choledochocanulophilia: Joy in having cannulated the bile duct during ERCP

Rajender K. Arora, MD, Orange, NJ

SILHOUETTIQUETTE

ASSIGNMENT:
Choose a feature on any map that resembles something in the medical spectrum.

EXAMPLES:
The former Czechoslovakia: The pancreas
Lake Michigan: The gallbladder
The Amazon watershed: A venous drainage system

ENTRIES:
Japan: Gastric peristalsis

> Melanio Villarosa, MD, Naples, FL

New Zealand: Otoscope

> Jayant Malhotra, MD, Homewood, IL

Central America: Side view of bladder and urethra

> Irving Thorne, MD, Minneapolis, MN

Italy: Phantom limb

> Betty Jung, Guilford, CT

The Grand Tetons: Knuckles

> Anthony Somkin, MD, Berkeley, CA

Japan: Peyronie's

> Dewey Heetderks, MD, Grand Rapids, MI

Florida: Terminal case of impotence and/or diabetes insipidus

> A. Somaskanda, MD, Sodus, NY

The Big Bend, Texas: A patient prepped for sigmoidoscopy

> Russell J. Cox, MD, Gastonia, NC

Norway and Sweden: Bifid uvula

> Charles G. Eschenburg, MD, Delray Beach, FL

New Guinea: A turkey that can't get off the ground, like government health care plan

Meyer B. Hodes, MD, Oceanside, NY

Aleutian Islands (upside down): Prostatic hypertrophy as seen on IVP

Morey Filler, MD, San Francisco, CA

Vietnam: Fallopian tube

Gene Westveer, MD, Zeeland, MI

Siberia (in a Mercator projection) Tongue's perception of a canker sore—lots larger than it really is

Marvin G. Gregory, MD, Nashville, TN

Nevis: Normal placenta
St. Kitts, Nevis's sister island: Battledore placenta (marginal cord insertion)

Julio Novoa, MD, Lutherville, MD

SAY IT AGAIN, SAM

ASSIGNMENT:
Fit a well-known person's quotation to a practice-related situation.

EXAMPLES:
Orthopedist Julius Caesar: "I came, I sawed, I conquered."

Gastroenterologist Ian Fleming: "Dangerous at both ends and uncomfortable in the middle."

Hospital administrator Mae West: "A man in the house is worth two in the street."

ENTRIES:
Beleaguered primary-care physician Marcus Tullius Cicero: "Oh what times! Oh what standards!"

Anthony J. Pierangelo, MD, Bonita, CA

Laser retinologist Colonel William Prescott: "Don't fire until you see the whites of their eyes."

Robert Ettlinger, MD, Dalmatia, PA

OB group obstetrician Lou Costello: "Who's on first; no, he's on second. What, he's on third."

David J. Schwartz, MD, Vineland, NJ

Pathologist George Bernard Shaw: "My specialty is being right when other people are wrong."

Neal Green, MD, Corsicana, TX

Orthopedist Don Herold (from a review of *Uncle Tom's Cabin*): "The dogs were poorly supported by the rest of the cast."

Morton F. Arnsdorf, MD, Chicago, IL

Epidemiologist Claude Rains: "Round up the usual suspects."

Melvin J. Breite, MD, Bayside, NY

Resuscitator Yogi Berra: "It ain't over till it's over."

Joseph F. J. Curi, MD, Torrington, CT

Housecall-seeking patient Mae West: "Why don't you come up and see me sometime?"

Gene Westveer, MD Zeeland, MI

Vascular surgeon Thomas Fuller: "Many little leaks can sink the ship."

Grafton C. Fanney, Jr., MD, Euclid, OH

Psychiatrist Yogi Berra: "It's déjà vu all over again."

Marvin G. Gregory, MD, Nashville, TN

Dermatologist Gerard Manley Hopkins: Glory be to God for dappled things."

Edward M. Sessa, MD, Schenectady, NY

JCAH inspector Arnold Schwarzenegger: "I'll be baaack!"

Russell J. Cox, MD, Gastonia, NC

THE MOMENT OF TRUTH

ASSIGNMENT:
How can a captive be made to talk using medical means?

EXAMPLES:
"You will be forced to watch a continuous slide show of histological specimens by a droning narrator. Sleep will be forbidden."

"You are, of course, familiar with this expandable Otis Urethrotome and its sliding blade . . ."

"A round-the-clock schedule of administrative meetings has been scheduled for you. No coffee . . ."

"They're icing down the flexible colonoscope right now . . ."

ENTRIES:
"Now that you've been prepped for a vasectomy, Dr. Parkinson will leave the room to get his L-DOPA."

Floyd T. Nasuti, MD, Philadelphia, PA

"First we inject the metal into various parts of your body. Then we begin the MRI scan."

Jeffrey Pearson, DO, San Marcos, CA

"We will endlessly clone your problem patients. They will never go away, never go away, never go away."

Marvin C. Gregory, MD, Nashville, TN

"Would you care to know just what the distance is from your incisors to your ileocecal valve?"

Melvin J. Breite, MD, Bayside, NY

"Congratulations. You've just been granted tenure on the Utilization Review Committee."

Neal Green, MD, Corsicana, TX

"Discharge the anesthetist and plug in the lithotripter . . ."

Morey Filler, MD, San Francisco, CA

"All the nurses you ever yelled at will use you to update their skills with nasogastric tubes, eighteen-gauge needles, and retention enemas."

Carlyn M. Kline, MD, St. Joseph, MO

"Okay, bring in the two-year-olds."

Susan E. Mahan, MD, Pueblo, CO

"You will be locked in an 8 x 12 foot exam room with an unbathed parent and a toddler with a dirty diaper until you respond."

Russell J. Cox, MD, Gastonia, NC

"Your last fifty admissions will be reviewed by a panel of discharge coordinators, malpractice lawyers, quality assurance managers, and managed-care coordinators."

Irving Thorne, MD, Mineapolis, MN

WITH FAINT PRAISE

ASSIGNMENT:
Tactfully convey a low opinion when asked for an evaluation.

EXAMPLES:
Q: "Would you take him as an associate?"
A: "It's too hypothetical. He's in a different specialty, which some say he practices adequately."
Q: "When she was in your locale, how was her clinical judgment?"
A: "She wasn't subject to any recent disciplinary action."
Q: "Was he a good partner?"
A: "He always picked up the tab at the Christmas party."

ENTRIES:
Q: "Is he an effective chief of service?"
A: "He will be a marvelous chairman emeritus."

Marvin G. Gregory, MD, Nashville, TN

Q: "Does he know how to handle complications?"
A: "Oh yes. I do not think there is a complication he has not seen."

Howard Landa, MD, Loma Linda, CA

Q: "Was the patient compliant with your instructions?"
A: "She always brought the correct child to the office."

Edward Lamon, MD, Albuquerque, NM

Q: "Was he a well-respected pathologist?"
A: "With few exceptions, I never heard a patient complain about him."

Edward M. Sessa, MD, Schenectady, NY

Q: "Did this physician complete a surgical residency at your institution?"
A: "Yes. He left the program well rested and in excellent health."

Robert B. Box, MD, Corbin, KY

Q: "Would you recommend this medical student for our residency?"
A: "He has a beautiful smile and is very popular with some of the nurses."

George T. Klauber, MD, Boston, MA

Q: "How were his surgical skills?"
A: "That's his greatest asset. You can still train him."

Neal Green, MD, Corsicana, TX

Q: "Would you let him operate on you?"
A: "I've already had my gall bladder removed."

Bernadine Z. Paulshock, Wilmington, DE

Q: "Are his progress notes complete and up-to-date?"
A: "He has beautiful handwriting."

J. Patrick Evans, MD, Savannah, GA

Morey Filler, MD, San Francisco, CA

MEDI-DOUBLESPEAK

ASSIGNMENT:
Create a lofty term for something commonplace.

EXAMPLES:
Oropharyngeal display system—tongue depressor
Health care facility vertical transportation engineer—hospital elevator operator
Reverse peristalsis product accumulator—emesis basin
Linear impetus propulsion provider—gurneyman

ENTRIES:
Saltatory conduction velocity estimator—reflex hammer
Deborah Erickson, MD, Hummelstown, PA

Portable tufted bipolar multifluid absorber—Q-tip
Robert R. Jones, MD, Nevada, MO

Digitalized graphic display chart documentation facilitator—pen
Lawrence W. Davis, MD, Riverside, CA

Manual self-contained hematologic retrieval system—syringe with needle
James R. Sevenich, MD, Stevens Point, WI

Esoteric cogitation promulgator—consultant
Stuart Cooperman, MD, Merrick, NY

Intermittent auditory or vibratory pleasure inhibitor—beeper
Margaret Bunger, MD, McLean, VA
Similarly, Russell J. Cox, MD, Gastonia, NC

Interim transition facility for thanatological investigation of the vitally challenged—morgue
Doris E. Fletcher, Kendall Park, NJ

Postpubertal confusional-confrontational dissonance syndrome—
adolescence

Ivan M. Safonoff, MD, New York, NY

Health care provider/consumer nonmechanical interface—receptionist

Pamela Chappen, Danville, PA

Muscular respiratory expulsion modifier solution—cough syrup

Neal Green, MD, Corsicana, TX

Multidiscipline health care provider convergence—hospital staff
meeting

J. Patrick Evans, MD, Savannah, GA

Elective/emergency provider/consumer hydration facility—hospital
water fountain

Cammie Eastham, Cincinnai, OH

Nocturnal marauder ova-sequestration readout—pinworm prep

John E. Daigre, Jr., MD, Lafayette, LA

THINGS THAT GO BUMP IN THE NIGHT

ASSIGNMENT:

Envision a medical nightmare at your door on Hallowe'en.

EXAMPLES:

Your PRO inquisitor carrying a history of charges in a bound volume.

The potential plaintiff who haunted your dreams, accompanied by a lawyer and papers, one week prior to the expiration of the statute of limitations.

A six-pack of new competitors paying a "courtesy call."

An OSHA SWAT team bearing blank checks for your signature.

ENTRIES:

An apologetic radiologist. He put the side marks backward on the IVP last week. And you did the nephrectomy this morning.

> Joel D. Lilly, MD, Seattle, WA

A family of encopretics in relapse.

> Russell J. Cox, MD, Gastonia, NC

A representative from the Yellow Pages mumbling something about your office number having been switched with the local massage parlor's.

> Jonathan S. Ehrlich, MD, Atlanta, GA

The 2,001 eight- to twelve-year-old girls under your care, all wanting to sell you Girl Scout cookies.

> Joseph F. J. Curi, MD, Torrington, CT

A new 386-pound hypertensive diabetic HMO patient, requesting a "complete checkup" as guaranteed by his contract.

> Jerome W. Lehrfeld, MD, Levittown, NY

Frankenstein, with a letter identifying you as his primary care doctor, wanting a face-lift.

Stan Hines, MD, Huntsville, TX

The ghosts of all your late patients saying that they miss you and want you to join their newly formed HMO.

Melvin J. Breite, MD, Bayside, NY

No fewer than two thousand HMO patients lined up, each counting out his $5 copayment in pennies.

Morey Filler, MD, San Francisco, CA

The Spirit of Enemas Past.

Neal Green, MD, Corsicana, TX

The lad on whom you did your first (after twelve tries) lumbar puncture, twenty years later—grown, wearing a hockey mask, and holding a chain saw.

Floyd T. Nasuti, MD, Philadelphia, PA

A patient from a capitation-based plan, carrying his head in a bag and stating that having been decapitated, he wishes recapitation.

E. M. Herrero, MD, Lincoln Park, MI

HOLD THAT LINE

ASSIGNMENT:

Program an answering machine message that endeavors to keep the doctor in bed.

EXAMPLES:

"If it's wet, dry it. If it's dry, wet it. If it itches, continue to scratch . . ." (Dermatologist)

"If you were able to see the dial to make this call, you're OK. If it had to be done for you, punch one for further instructions." (Ophthalmologist)

ENTRIES:

"You have reached the office of Dr. Finetune. If your funding is with I&D HMO, enter the first twenty digits of the number at the top of your card. If this is a workers' compensation claim, press star if you're willing to sign an affidavit that your injury is legitimate. If you're insured with Capitation Care, press the pound sign to select your musical preference. If you're on Medicaid, your call did not go through. Please hang up and dial again."

Anthony Somkin, MD, Berkeley, CA

"We have been hooked up to a 900 number. Conversation is twenty-five dollars a minute. Insurance coverage does not apply. Have your charge card number handy and stay on the line."

Bernadine Z. Paulshock, MD, Wilmington, DE

"If this message lasts longer than you did, call us in the morning." (Impotence clinic)

Jeffrey Pearson, DO, San Marcos, CA

"If you know who you are and the time you are calling, hang up and call us in the morning." (Neurologist)

Edward M. Sessa, MD, Poughkeepsie, NY

Venereal clinic: "Take two aspirin and stay out of bed for a few days."

Carl Sorgen, MD, Poughkeepsie, NY

ER physician: "If you know you're ill or hurt, press one. If you suspect you're ill or hurt, press two. If you wonder if you're ill or hurt, press three. If you pressed one, two, or three, you will reach four, which will automatically dial a board-certified psychiatrist who will assist you in the resolution of your conflict. When you are comfortable with your condition, please call back. If you are calling back, press five. Five will get you six that you will be better by morning."

Hugh H. Wang, MD, Clayton, CA

Dermatologist: "If you have a rash, please photograph it now so when you get to the office, I can tell you what you have."

M. David Lauter, MD, York, ME

Pulmonologist: "At the tone, exhale forcefully. We will automatically calculate your peak flow and adjust your asthma medications."

Margriet Bunger, MD, McLean, VA

SHADES OF DIFFERENCE

ASSIGNMENT:

Show how use of the first, second, and third persons can express the subtleties of bias.

EXAMPLES:

"I performed a difficult phlebotomy; you searched for a vein; he/she struck repeatedly."

"I treat vigorously; you treat adequately; he/she overprescribes!"

"I did a digital exam; you poked; he/she ramrodded."

"I made a surgical decision; you made a judgment call; he/she was quick to operate."

ENTRIES:

"I palpate. You feel. He/she gropes."

Peter A. DeGregorio, MD, Scottsdale, AZ

"I detected the subtle murmur. You thought you heard something. He/she said, "It's a heart.""

Morey Filler, MD, San Francisco, CA

"I did a multilayered plastic repair. You sutured a wound. He/she sewed up a gash."

Jerome W. Lehrfeld, MD, Levittown, NY

"I got a second opinion on that obscure call. You checked before making a commitment. He/she ought to have Mayo on retainer."

Patricia Barwig, MD, Wauwatosa, WI

"I close abdomens beautifully. Did you invent the zigzag stitch? He/she has distilled the essence of dehiscence."

Ivan M. Safonoff, MD, New York, NY

"I spend cognitive time with patients. You take too long. He/she lets the schedule bog down."

Jeffery J. Rabinovitz, MD, Placerville, CA

"I position. You manipulate. He/she cranks."

James A. Krug, MD, Placerville, CA

"I expanded my intellectual database. You had to get some CMEs. He/she required remedial instruction.

Joseph B. Szgalsly, MD, Woodbury, NJ

"I am of the Osler tradition. You are well grounded in the basics. He/she—well, even a blind hog will find an acorn now and then.

Stan Hines, MD, Huntsville, TX

"I made some fee miscalculations. You overcharged. He/she robbed the public blind."

John A. Conti, MD, New York, NY

"On hearing hoofbeats, I think horses; you, zebras; he/she, eagles.

Anthony Somkin, MD, Berkeley, CA

TOMFOOLERY

ASSIGNMENT:

Create a statement so preposterous that a postscript—"April Fool!"—would be a mere formality.

EXAMPLES:

"We at Medicare feel you were undercompensated. Enclosed is a check . . ."

"Our PRO office was overzealous. Accept our apologies for your trouble and this stipend for your time and mileage."

Letter to hospital administrator from nearby hospital: "We congratulate you on the acquisition of your new equipment. Since the community will benefit thereby, we'll cancel our plans to acquire it and use your facility . . ."

"Because you are the 10,000th patient to pass through our portals, all expenses for your hospital stay will be waived."

ENTRIES:

"An anonymous physician has agreed to take your night calls for the remainder of the year."

Russell J. Cox, MD, Gastonia, NC

To OB patient from insurance company: "We understand you weren't well enough to go home the day after your delivery. Please stay in the hospital until you feel well. We'll take care of the bill."

Alan Goldman, MD, Raleigh, NC

Sign in front of hospital emergency room: THOSE WHO COME HERE FOR TRUE EMERGENCIES WILL BE TREATED FREE.

S. Bharath, MD, Devil's Lake, ND

"Thank you for treating my cough, Doctor. Since I know how valuable your time is, I'll schedule another appointment to discuss my mood swings."

Leland J. Davis, MD, Santa Rosa, CA

"In that you were the millionth colonoscopy patient in our center, your prep and procedure were taped to be seen nationwide on a leading talk show."

Kenneth A. Deitcher, MD, Albany, NY

"Doctor, please, may I pay my entire surgical fee in advance, in cash?"

Catherine Sladowski, MD Verona, NJ

"Hospital quarterly staff meetings will now be held annually. Sign-ins by voice mail are permissible."

Edward M. Sessa, MD, Schenectady, NY

Memo from state capital: "Due to its dreaded nature, all paperwork hereby is considered illegal in this state and should be discontinued ASAP. Destroy this memo immediately to maintain compliance."

Pamela Chappen, Danville, PA

From malpractice carrier: "Because you have not been involved in any litigation for the past ten years, you may disregard this premium notice."

Andrew C. Feldman, DO, DeLand, FL

GEOMEDRY

ASSIGNMENT:
Associate a medical trait that is characteristic of the name of an area, place, or region.

EXAMPLES:
Valsalvador: Where bearing down is everything

Semipalatinsk (Kazakstan): Where the oral surgeon is constantly challenged

Eukrainium: Where no substitute exists for a good head

The Peereknees: Where arthroscopy is at its highest level

ENTRIES:
Santa Fe: Home of the patron saint of hemochromatosis
> Floyd T. Nasuti, MD, Philadelphia, PA

Constantinibble: Bulimia treatment center
> Ralph French, MD, Anna Maria, FL

Slingapore: The birthplace of dermatological orthopedics
> Philip S. Green, MD, Piscataway, NJ

Watemala: Where tourists are cautioned against drinking from wells
> E. U. Herrero, MD, Lincoln Park, MI

South Bends: Austral region hazardous to scuba divers
> Alex Krammer, MD, Covina, CA

Subluxembourg: Dey got a big orthopedic joint in dis location
> Ivan M Safonoff, MD, New York, NY

Kinchow: Where potassium depletion is never a problem
> Doris E. Fletcher, Kendall Park, NJ

Oslo: Uterine prolapse capital of the world
> Jonathan S. Ehrlich, MD, Atlanta, GA

Jim-Bob's Way: A surgical approach popular in old Southern Rhodesia

Charles G. Eschenburg, MD, Atlanta, GA

Khartomb: Where Dr. Kevorkian discharges his Detroit patients

Jeffrey Pearson, DO, San Marcos, CA

Pawtucket: Future site of the geriatric male abdominoplasty research center

Marvin G. Gregory, MD, Nashville, TN

Vicksburg: Center for holistic pulmonology

Edward M. Sessa, MD, Schenectady, NY

Moretaenia: Where thrives a large tapeworm population

Alan Goldman, MD, Raleigh, NC

Etheropia: Sanctuary for elderly, visually impaired anesthesiologists

Robert R. Jones, MD, Nevada, MO

Bursalona: Location of 1992 Summer Olympics, vulnerable to flare-ups.

Sylvia Bernstein, Far Rockaway, NY

HAVING HAD IT

ASSIGNMENT:

In stating that a practitioner is "over the hill," devise a specialty-specific way of saying, "Dr. X's career is . . ."

EXAMPLES:

". . . red cells in the sunset."—Hematologist
". . . chopped liver."—Pathologist
". . . down the tubes."—Gynecologist
". . . past history."—Medical record librarian

ENTRIES:

". . . out to Pasteur."—Bacteriologist

Philip Paul, MD, Miami, FL

". . . down for the count."—Hematologist

Laura A. B. Cifelli, Flemington, NJ

". . . belly-up."—General surgeon

Walton D. Bailey, Jr., MD, Bryan, TX

". . . played-out."—Pediatrician

Dan MacDougall, MD, Renton, WA

". . . dormant."—Anesthesiologist

Eugenia P. Lantz, MD, Ft. Lauderdale, FL

". . . flat-lined."—Cardiologist

Richard J. Gimpelson, MD, Chesterfield, MO

". . . at the 'Y.'"—Pathologist

Joseph G. Richardson, MD, Rochester, MN

". . . run its course."—Sports medicine

Gerald S. Roberts, MD, Lake Success, NY

"... water under the bridge."—Urologist

Joseph B. Szgalsky, MD, Woodbury, NJ

"... over and out."—Flight surgeon

J. Xavier Castillo, MD, Pomona, CA

"... up in smoke."—Laser surgeon

Elaine Schwab, Albany, NY

"... losing power."—EEG technician

Charles G. Eschenburg, MD, Delray Beach, FL

"... flown the Koop."—Surgeon general

Doris M. Cowley, MD, Bryan, TX

"... off the charts."—Medical records

Norman D. Lindley, MD, Alamogordo, NM

"... ready for the fat lady to sing."—Endocrinologist

Gary J. Coomber, MD, Santa Rosa, CA

"... returned to the dust whence it came."—Allergist

Marvin G. Gregory, MD, Nashville, TN

"... on the rocks."—Lithotripser

Burnell Stripling, MD, Marinette, WI

"... sagging woefully."—Plastic surgeon

Neal Green, MD, Corsicana, TX

"... in withdrawal and shrinking fast."—Psychiatrist

Ivan M. Safonoff, MD, New York, NY

"... grown long in the tooth."—Dentist

Jerome W. Lehrfeld, MD, Levittown, NY

". . . getting ready to blow the joint."—Orthopedist

Hugh Wang, MD, Clayton, CA

". . . no code."—Geneticist

Jonathan S. Ehrlich, MD, Atlanta, GA

". . . incapable of being maintained."—Urologist

Carlyn M. Kline, MD, St. Joseph, MO

". . . fallen and unable to get up."—Gerontologist

Ronald H. Smalley, MD, Flint, MI

ACTA OPERATICA

ASSIGNMENT:
Alter an opera title and plot in a medical way.

EXAMPLES:
Wrigletto: Heroic neurologist cures an epidemic of purposeless movements.

Götterdämmerol: A villainous elf holds the key to the kingdom's narcotics. It is wrenched from him by means of a persuasion device, the wring cycle.

The Magic Fruit: A gallant gastroenterologist, a retirement community, and prunes.

Ill Trovatore: An ailing troubador is finally cured after a cameo appearance by an ambulance-based heroine physician, la Donna Mobile.

ENTRIES:
The Threepenny Operation: A grasping, numismatic thoracic surgeon seeks to extract several coin lesions of the lung. To his dismay, these prove to be worthless artifacts as a result of pulmonary hyperinflation.

Joseph Grayzel, MD, Englewood, NJ

Done One: The middle volume of an operatic trilogy on medical education. Its prequel is Saw One, and its sequel is Taught One. Contains the famous aria "Vesti la Scrubba."

Anatoly Belilovsky, MD, Brooklyn, NY

La behemoth: A morbidly obese French girl's search for a diet ends tragically when, mistaking the white-coated bariatrician for a marshmallow, she eats him.

Jonathan S. Ehrlich, MD, Atlanta, GA

La Send the Rent Over: The story of negotiations between the HMO and the office complex management.

Candace S. Whitehurst, MD, Norfolk, VA

The Lying Dutchman: A notorious case of Münchausen syndrome is doomed to roam the hospital corridors of the world for eternity unless he can marry a Korsakoff's psychotic and lie with her happily ever after.

Ivan M. Safonoff, MD, New York, NY

Un Ballo en Mascara: A talented plastic surgeon perfects permanent eye makeup.

Carlyn M. Kline, MD, St. Joseph, MO

Signor Butterfly: A young surgeon meets antagonism from the old guard as he tries to introduce a new method of closing skin incisions. Highlight is the poignant "Steri-Strip" aria.

Jerome W. Lehrfeld, MD, Levittown, NY

Trotska: An opera-ballet in which Montezuma gets even in Russia, teaching Russians the two-step.

Ralph French, MD, Anna Maria, FL

Lab O'Heme: A group of technicians in a Left Bank garret struggle, live, and die. Ironically, the heroine, Anemi, succumbs to RBC depletion.

Gary J. Coomber, MD, Santa Rosa, CA

Thighs: The tragic story of a plastic surgeon who is allergic to the cellulite he removes. His Act I finale, "Lipo Not for Mio." leaves not a dry eye in the audience.

Franklin L. Brosgol, MD, Chappaqua, NY

Tanninghouser: A sinister dermatologist lures unsuspecting clients to a tanning salon where they develop skin cancer for which they require his treatment.

Norman D. Lindley, MD, Alamogordo, NM

The Marriage of Figuro: An Italian plastic surgeon perfects liposuction in his small town and, prospering, wins the hand of his inamorata.

A. Morris, Dickson City, PA

Romeo and Joliet: Despicable lothario who bilks older women goes from their life savings to his life sentence after being nabbed by a transvestite undercover agent.

Dr. Louis DiBacco, Aldan, PA

Modem Butterfly: Overenthusiastic doc goes online, develops lupus-like eruption as part of Overuse syndrome.

John Glennon, MD, Granville, NY

Ahnal and the Night Visitors: A young boy is pestered by chronic pinworm infestations.

Jeffrey Pearson, DO, San Marcos, CA

Madama Butterfat: B. F. Pinkerton, bariatric internist extraordinaire, fights to save his beloved geisha, Oh Li Oh Butterfat, from terminal obesity, brought on by the loneliness of his long absence. Another fat chance for the good doctor!

Charles W. Webb, MD, Owosso, MI

ER TO THE FAMOUS

ASSIGNMENT:
Treat a prominent person with a prominent affliction as you would any emergency room walk-in.

EXAMPLES:
"Pectoral pruritus is no emergency, Monsieur Bonaparte. Here's an appointment for the dermatology clinic."

"He's a whaleboat skipper with an outdated prosthesis."

"We got this snakebit queen off the river."

"You say you're a painter? Well sit down with your ear and wait your turn."

ENTRIES:
"The ophthalmologist on call will be in to check her soon, Mr. Warbucks."

A. E. Mgebroff, MD, Yoakum, TX

"Will Rogers is here with a rectal abscess, and he doesn't want to meet the ER physician."

Louis DeBacco, DO, Aldan, PA

"That's a strange-looking burn, Mr. Roentgen. Have you any idea what caused it?"

Marvin G. Gregory, MD, Nashville, TN

"He's a German preacher who just hit his thumb with a hammer."

Carlyn M. Kline, MD, St. Joseph, MO

"Doctor, Mr. Buckley here says he can't move to his left."

H. K. Bunnell, MD, Soda Springs, ID

"We can't give you a prescription for anabolic steroids just because you had a haircut."

Gene Westveer, MD, Zeeland, MI

"We have this gunslinging dentist with a bad cough."

Jeffrey R. Scott, MD, Englewood, CO

"Immediate social work referral for a forty-five-year-old mother of twenty, in need of a home due to a narrow toe box."

Ellen San Buenaventura, MD, Tucson, AZ

"No wonder you can't breathe. Your corset is too tight, Miss Scarlett."

Bernadine Z. Paulshock, MD, Wilmington, DE

"There's some old guy out here dressed in a sheet, with a fiddle and second-degree burns."

J. Patrick Evans, MD, Savannah, GA

"I know your son has trouble walking, Mr. Cratchit, but right now he just ate too much Christmas dinner."

William R. Coyle, MD, Fort Washington, MD

"He is asking for a vet to treat the frostbite on his elephant's feet.

Charles G. Eschenburg, MD, Delray Beach, FL

IN THE BEGINNING

ASSIGNMENT:
In a specialty-specific way, describe the beginning of one's career, beginning with, "Dr. X's career is . . ."

EXAMPLES:
". . . embryonic."—Obstetrician
". . . infantile."—Pediatrician
". . . first seeing the light of day."—Ophthalmologist
". . . pre-carious."—Dentist

ENTRIES:
". . . antediluvian."—Urologist

Edward M. Thompson, MD, Dillsburg, PA

". . . still in the starting blocks."—Anesthesiologist

Lewis Shilane, DO, Joplin, MO

". . . prehysteric."—Psychiatrist

Alan L. Goldman, MD, Raleigh, NC

". . . coming out of the shadows."—Sonographer

Julio Novoa, MD, Lutherville, MD

". . . finally trained."—Pediatrician

Forrest P. White, MD, Norfolk, VA

". . . ballooning."—Invasive cardiologist.

Doris M. Cowley, MD, College Station, TX

". . . beginning to perk."—Hospital administrator

Walton D. Bailey, Jr., MD, College Station, TX

". . . undergoing pollination."—Allergist

Melanio P. Villarosa, MD, Naples, FL

". . . still in the process of getting pre-appraised."—HMO medical director

Barry Bzostek, MD, Fort Worth, TX

". . . at the portal."—Hepatologist.

Melvin J. Breite, MD, Bayside, NY

". . . beginning descent."—Pediatric urologist

Philip A. Batista, MD, Indianapolis, IN

". . . at stage I."—Oncologist

Joseph F. J. Curi, MD, Torrington, CT

". . . myelocytic."—Hematologist

Jerome W. Lehrfeld, MD, Levittown, NY

". . . prehensile."—Hand surgeon

Earl J. Carstensen, MD, Denver, CO

". . . catching on."—Epidemiologist

Sylvia Bernstein, Far Rockaway, NY

DR. BFTSPLK

ASSIGNMENT:
Patterned after Al Capp's beclouded character who brought catastrophic misfortune wherever he went, create a doctor who treads the health care landscape with similar havoc in his wake. As he passes . . . .

EXAMPLES:
. . . the OR, the bearer slips on K-Y jelly, precipitating the donor organ against the surgeon's spectacles.

. . . the pathology lab, the rado emits a freqency high enough to shatter one thousand slides.

. . . the annual hospital Christmas party, a jar of diuretic tablets overturns on a shelf, spilling its contents into the punch bowl, where they dissolve.

. . . the groundbreaking ceremonies for a hospital addition, the orator, in midspeech, is suddenly afflicted with Tourette's syndrome.

ENTRIES:
. . . *an emergency laparoscopy*, the patient has to be removed from the ceiling because the nurse has mistakenly substituted a tank of helium for one of CO_2.

Julio Novoa, MD, Lutherville, MD

. . . *the OR scheduling office*, the computer sticks and prints "8:00 AM, Room 10" on all thirty of the next morning's surgery cases."

Alan L. Goldman, MD, Raleigh, NC

. . . *the office*, the sharps containers explode and hazardous waste hits the fan during an inspection by the OSHA man.

Ivan M. Safonoff, MD, New York, NY

. . . *the Respiratory Therapy Unit*, all the incentive spirometry patients become synchronized, causing the room to implode.

Marvin G. Gregory, MD, Nashville, TN

. . . the hospital switchboard, the page operator leaves the switch open as she gossips about the liaison between the Chief of Surgery and the Director of Nurses.

Donald Barkan, MD, Swampscott, MA

. . . the imaging suite, the barium enema catheter is attached to the positive pressure ventilator.

Charles G. Eschenburg, MD, Delray Beach, FL

. . . the EKG Department, all tracings suddenly show nonspecific S-T changes, not just the usual 80%.

Richard H. Morris, MD, Harrison, OH

. . . the athletic field house, the sports medicine specialist, having spilled muscle ointment balm into the Preparation H jar, is chased out of town by eleven angry men.

Neal Green, MD, Corsicana, TX

SO TO SPEAK

ASSIGNMENT:
Associate a well-known catchphrase with a medical situation.

EXAMPLES:
He has been known to do a craniotomy at the drop of a hat.
Heel surgery was done on the spur of the moment.
Blepharitis was diagnosed in the blink of an eye.
He won the race for ENT department chairman by a nose.

ENTRIES:
They tried family planning after six of one, half a dozen of the other.

Dan MacDougall, Mercer Island, WA

The diabetic found the fingerprick method short, sweet, and to the point.

J. Malhotra, MD, Homewood, IL

The Mohs surgeon passed his boards by the narrowest of margins.

Ronald P. Spencer, MD, Ocala, FL

The very idea of genetic engineering drove him up a tree.

Carlyn M. Kline, MD, St. Joseph, MO

Results of the gastric stapling-laryngoplasty won't be known till the fat lady sings.

Lewis Shilane, DO, Joplin, MO

The physiatrist got his back up at the thought of the Stryker frame.

James P. McCann, MD, Wabash, IN

His gastroscopy was canceled because he didn't have the stomach for it.

A. N. Feinberg, MD, Kalamazoo, MI

They all chewed the fat at the liposuction workshop.

Laurie Clark, DO, Tulsa, OK

Environmental control is nothing to sneeze at.

Brendan Duterte, MD, Santa Clara, CA

I'm going to give that neurosurgeon a piece of my mind!

Anne Simons, San Francisco, CA

The hematologist, rheumatologist, and ophthalmologist enjoyed the performance of Blood, Sweat & Tears.

Malcolm Phillips, MD, Great Neck, NY

After blepharoplasties and gastric stapling, his eyes were bigger than his stomach.

Marvin G. Gregory, MD, Nashville, TN

We thought he was a good lithotripser, but he turned out to be just a flash in the pan.

Ivan M. Safonoff, MD, New York, NY

He does cervical laminectomies at breakneck speed.

Neal Green, MD, Corsicana, TX

The pacemaker was inserted just under the wire.

Donald Barkan, MD, Swampscott, MA

TOUGH LUCK

ASSIGNMENT:

Envision a medical situation in which the disastrous and the wondrous dovetail.

EXAMPLES:

A fire destroys the block containing your office and that of the lawyer housing your malpractice suit papers.

Having been enriched by your sale of land, you learn that it is to be the site of a clinic housing six competitors.

All your medical organizations' dues have been waived because of your age.

ENTRIES:

You are the local expert in a procedure that everyone refers to you, but it is "experimental." All payers decline reimbursement.

Hugh H. Wang, MD, Clayton, CA

Your heroic feats saved a premature infant who grew up to become the leader of an underground terrorist organization.

Russell J. Cox, MD, Gastonia, NC

Your physician encourages you to continue smoking, as it is already too late to quit.

Karl J. Pizzolato, MD, Baton Rouge, LA

Hospital security reports that your missing beeper has turned up at the pediatric clinic—in the waiting room aquarium.

Joseph F. J. Curi, MD, Torrington, CT

You get your first choice on Internship Match Day. However, the computer made a slight error on "Cedars of Lebanon Hospital," and you're off to Beirut.

Alan L. Goldman, MD, Raleigh, NC

Your patient with hypertension and priapism does not experience side effects from his effective antihypertensive medicine.

Richard H. Morris, MD, Harrison, OH

You are cited for giving "the breath of life" to a Code Blue patient, only to learn he succumbed to drug-resistant M. tuberculosis.

Burnell Stripling, MD, Marinette, WI

Your malpractice attorney notifies you that his rates are discounted after the fifth case.

Anthony John Battista, Stewart Manor, NY

Your son's school phobia is cured. Now he refuses to leave school.

Charles G. Eschenburg, MD, Delray Beach, FL

You give your only daughter the wedding of her dreams, welcoming into the family the son of a patient who successfully sued you for "wrongful birth."

Carlyn M. Kline, MD, St. Joseph, MO

An employee is found to have been skimming the profits, but he's kept accurate records of all thefts and invested wisely.

Grafton C. Fanney, MD, Euclid, OH

IN PRIME RHYME

ASSIGNMENT:

Substitute two rhymed words for two nonrhyming ones in the medical domain.

EXAMPLES:

Curt caregiver = Terse nurse
Craving for colloids = Emulsion compulsion
Catgut's successor = Future suture
The pregnancy imperative = Gravidity avidity
Stretcherperson of average skills = Journeyman gurneyman

ENTRIES:

Hirsute blisters = Woolly bullae

Wilmot S. McCullough III, MD, Sumter, SC

Submental liposuction specimen jar = Wattle bottle.

Marvin G. Gregory, MD, Nashville, TN

Dilantin doubter = Skeptic epileptic

Ivan M. Safonoff, MD, NYC, NY

Enigmatic psychiatrists = Sphinx shrinks

Barnaby Starr, MD, Baltimore, MD

Tendon Neurosis = Achilles willies

Robert Flora, MD, Putnam Valley, NY

Neuroanatomical nemesis = Ridiculous fasciculus

Jerome W. Lehrfeld, MD, Levittown, NY

Glutei = Bustle muscle

Sidney G. Piness, MD, Plainfield, NJ

Histology journal = Tissue issue

Lewis Shilane, DO, Joplin, MO

Reputed mass = Tumor rumor

Hugh H. Wang, MD, Clayton, CA

Laparoscopic gallbladder removal = Holey choly

Alan M. Wagner, MD, Glendale, WI

Allergic reaction = Mast blast

Russell J. Cox, MD, Gastonia, NC

Icteric specialty society inductee = Yellow fellow

Barry L. Shickman, MD, San Antonio, TX

Trismus = Tight bite

R. J. Lindeman, MD, Paynesville, MN

Artificial liver blueprint = Hepatic schematic

Richard L. Dermody, MD, Breese, IL

Anemia = Inadequate hematocrit

David M. Pollack, MD, Swarthmore, PA

Czech composer's eye layers = Smetana's retinas

Sylvia Bernstein, Far Rockaway, NY

Laplanders' genitalia = Nomads' gonads

Morey Filler, MD, San Francisco, CA

Relief bottle of formula = Lactation vacation

Floyd T. Nasuti, MD, Philadelphia, PA

Diverticulum = Hole in colon

Melvin J. Breite, MD, Bayside, NY

Invaders' care facility = Insurgency emergency

M. B. Hanson, MD, Fort Thomas, KY

Ganglion = wrist cyst

Arthur N. Feinberg, MD, Kalamazoo, MI

Obstetrician from New Mexico = Adobe OB

Charles G. Eschenburg, MD, Delray Beach, FL

Transplant transporter = Liver quiver

Morey Filler, MD, San Francisco, CA

False evidence in malpractice trial = Surgery perjury

Meyer Hodes, MD, East Rockaway, NY

Cigarette smoker = Cancer chancer

Michelle Taube, MD, Hana, HI

Manipulating oncogenes = Cancer's answers

John A. Conti, MD, New York, NY

Impotence surgery = Erection correction

Richard J. Gimpelson, MD, Chesterfield, MO

Most knowledgeable PRO staffer = Review guru

Robert R. Jones, MD, Nevada, MO

DR. PRIMROSE

ASSIGNMENT:
Ogden Nash's absentminded Mr. Primrose transposed his actions. Envision what a medical person might do (i.e., "He frequently lit his hair and combed his cigar." Or "He tipped his students and flunked the traffic policeman") with such a stigma upon him.

EXAMPLES:
He scrubbed the specimen and labeled his hands . . . nibbled on a hemostat and autoclaved his lunch . . . submitted some blades and needles and tossed the insurance forms into the sharps container . . . hung up the blistered foot and punctured the IV bag.

ENTRIES:
. . . folded the patient and turfed the wheelchair.
Carlyn M. Kline, MD, St. Joseph, MO

. . . bandaged the OR nurse and thanked the patient
Vito E. Caselnova, MD, Babylon, NY

. . . delivered the flowers and watered the baby.
Morey Filler, MD, San Francisco, CA

. . . sent the chart to X-ray and put the patient back in the rack.
Marvin G. Gregory, MD, Nashville, TN

. . . increased the traction and reduced his fee.
H. Wesley Brown, MD, Mentor, OH

. . . billed the consultant and queried the patient.
Jerome W. Lehrfeld, MD, Levittown, NY

. . . (tired intern) sipped the light and turned off his soda.
Joseph A. Troncale, MD, New Holland, PA

. . . telemonitored his lunch and microwaved the pacemaker.
Donald Barkan, MD, Swampscott, MA

. . . set the fracture and reset the pulse.

Edward Thompson, MD, Mechanicsburg, PA

. . . took a specimen from the blood agar plate and incubated the child for overnight growth.

Alan L. Goldman, MD, Raleigh, NC

. . . immunized the balloons and blew up the children.

Florence Glazer, Yonkers, NY

. . . auscultated the Pap slide and smeared the chest.

Lillian Kinsey, PA, Lexington, KY

. . . peered into a polyp and snared a colonoscope.

Michael R. Cohen, MD, Petersburg, VA

MOVING THE QUESTION

ASSIGNMENT:
Given an answer, provide the medical question that elicited it.

EXAMPLES:
A: A eustacian wagon.
Q: What type of car takes ENT patients to the hospital?

A: Sacreligious.
Q: How do you describe a bursal or scrotal fanatic?

A: A rhizotomy.
Q: What did the neurosurgeon get when he described my imminent operation?

A: Ossicles.
Q: What is ice hanging from the earlobes?

ENTRIES:
A: Small deposits and early withdrawals.
Q: How does a banker describe male infertility?
Neal Green, MD, Corsicana, TX

A: Equilibrium.
Q: What do horses take for anxiety?
Anatoly Belilovsky, MD, Brooklyn, NY

A: Osteoblast
Q: What do you call a skeletons' party?
Grafton C. Fanney, Jr., MD, Euclid, OH

A: The eyelets of Langerhans.
Q: What's taking Brinker so long to lace up his ice skates?
James A. Canfield, MD, New York, NY

A: The auricle at Delphi.
Q: What fortune-teller has a lovely seaside home with a nice atrium?
Ivan M. Safonoff, MD, New York, NY

A: Metastatic.

Q: What does the oncologist complain of when using a cellular phone?

Doris E. Fletcher, MD, Kendall Park, NJ

A: Islet cell.

Q: Where was the sugar thief imprisoned?

Joseph Grayzel, MD, Englewood, NJ

A: Colectomy.

Q: How does a mother tell her college-bound son to call?

Edward M Thompson, MD, Dillsburg, PA

A: Café au lait spots.

Q: Where do teetotaling residents hang out after hours?

Russell J. Cox, MD, Gastonia, NC

A: Bundle of His.

Q: What's she suing him for?

David M. Cameron, MD and Thomas M. Evans,
MD, Cincinnati, OH

A: Amenorrhea.

Q: What is an overflowing end-of-prayer approval?

Michael R. Cohen, MD, Petersburg, VA

A: Borborygmi.

Q: What small-statured African tribe speaks an odd language of rumbles and gurgles?

D. Eric Tutt, MD, Mesa, AZ

A: Officiate.

Q: What caused the angler's gastroenteritis?

M. David Lauter, MD, York, ME

A: Carcinoid.

Q: What does Jay Leno aspire to be?

Kenneth G. Davis, MD, Conroe, TX

THE TWAIN SHALL MEET

ASSIGNMENT:
Name a corporate entity combining a doctor's practice and outside business.

EXAMPLES:
The Catcher in the Rye: Obstetrician / liquor retailer
The Bries and Eye: Cheese merchant / ophthalmologist
Hide and Seek: Dermatologist / private detective

ENTRIES:
See Spot Run: Ophthalmologist / dry cleaner
> Mazhar Elamir, MD, Jersey City, NJ

Fryer Tuck: Short-order cook / plastic surgeon
> M. David Lauter, MD, York, ME

Shake and Bake: Neurologist / pastry chef
> Christopher R. Morris, MD, Kingsport, TN

Shrinking Violet: Psychiatrist / florist
> Floyd T. Nasuti, MD, Philadelphia, PA

Ticker Tape: Cardiologist / recording artist
> Neal Green, MD, Corsicana, TX

Cough and Trough: Pulmonologist / hog farmer
> Charles G. Eschenburg, MD, Delray Beach, FL

Hackandsack: Pulmonologist / grocer
> Russell J. Cox, MD, Gastonia, NC

Field and Stream: Farmer / urologist
> Allan G. Plaut, MD, Lawrence, NY

Ova and Parasites: Fertility expert / law firm
> Irving Thorne, MD, St. Louis Park, MN

A BUN in the Oven: Nephrologist / baker

Donna R. Potruch, RN, West Hills, CA

Rank and File: Appraiser / podiatrist

Joseph F. J. Curi, MD, Torrington, CT

Bump and Grind: Acne specialist / lens maker

Alan L. Goldman, Raleigh, NC

Chateauneuf-du-Pap: Vintner / cytopathologist

Joseph Grayzel, MD, Englewood, NJ

Pees and Cues: Urologist / actor

Carlyn Kline, MD, St. Joseph, MO

Straighten Up and Fly Right: Orthopedist / travel agent

Melvin J. Breite, MD, Bayside, NY

Ribs R Us: Specialty restauranteur / thoracic surgeon

Jerome W. Lehrfeld, MD, Levittown, NY

Arsenic and Old Lace: Toxicologist / antiques dealer

Charles W. Webb, MD, Owosso, MI

Fore Your Eyes Only: Ophthalmologist / golf pro

Lisa Shakerin, MD, Crystal, MN

The Achin' Knee and the Acts to See: Orthopedic surgeon / talent agent

Jonathan Kurland, MD, Orinda, CA

The Gooed, the Bared, and the Ugly: Pediatrician / photographer's model / IRS agent

Jonathan S. Ehrlich, MD, Atlanta, GA

DOCTOR DOCKERS

ASSIGNMENT:
Christen boats with names that reflect doctor' interests.

EXAMPLES:
The Sea Arm—Radiologist
Surface Phenomenon—Dermatologist
Aquatic Quadruped—A four-pediatrician group

ENTRIES:
Windjammer—Gastroenterologist

William O. Ameen, Jr., MD, Greensboro, NC

Bowman's Capsule—Nephrologist

Rick Hiller, MD, Houston, TX

V-Tack—Five-cardiologist group

Lawrence K. Harris, MD, Reading, PA

To See Seas—Pharmacist

Michael Ichniowski, MD, Lutherville, MD

Dr. Doolittle—Retired MD

Robert L. Hillery, MD, Findlay, OH

Sailbad the Sinner—Substance abuse specialist

Willis L. Dixon, MD, East Grand Rapids, MI

Pequod—Four-man urology group

Arthur Montagne, MD, Manchester, CT

Aquaknot—Surgeon

Barnaby Starr, MD, Baltimore, MD

Triream—Urologist

R. M. Kniseley, MD, Oak Ridge, TN

Jolly Rongeur—Neurosurgeon

> Daniel K. Jass, MD, Lawrenceville, NJ

Rheum and Starboard—Arthrologist

> David H. Bisharat, Seattle, WA

Elbowtross—Orthopedist

> Miles Klein, Asbury Park, NJ

Three Sheets to the Wind—Anesthesiologist

> Sabrina Mentock, MD, Durham, NC

Sea Pap—Intensivist

> Gordon Hutcheon, Teaneck, NJ

Bay Window—Bariatrician

> Thomas R. White, MD, St. Petersburg, FL

Fissureman—Proctologist

> Susanne Latessa, R.N., Sterling Heights, MI

Pier Pressure—Psychologist

> Sylvia Bernstein, Far Rockaway, NY

Bottom Slapper—Obstetrician

> Michael D. Horn, MD, Cherry Hill, NJ

Channel Blocker—Cardiologist

> Grafton C. Fanney, Jr., MD, Euclid, OH

Anchors Aweigh—Locum tenens

> Robert M. Pickoff, MD, Somerset, NJ

Graft Craft—Plastic surgeon

> Raul A. Estrada, MD, Newport Beach, CA

Vara Seas—Gastroenterologist

> Nancy O'Bryan, RN, Owensboro, KY

Hard A Tack—Cardiologist

Dr. Henry Ruehle, Houston, TX

King of the Seize—Neurologist

Ivan Safonoff, MD, New York, NY

OSHAnographer—Safety inspector

Alan L. Goldman, MD, Raleigh, NC

My T-Wave—Cardiologist

Donald Barkan, MD, Swampscott, MA

The Amnionaut—Obstetrician

Julio Novoa, MD, Lutherville, MD

Lazy I—Ophthalmologist

Lillian E. Chin, MD, Philadelphia, PA

Normal Saline—ER physician

James P. McCann, MD, Wabash, IN

Il Pisscatore—Urologist

Daniel Schual-Berke, MD, Seattle, WA

MALAPROPERLY SPEAKING

ASSIGNMENT:
Malaprop a well-known phrase, word, title, or expression into the medical sphere.

EXAMPLES:
This is one of our hardiest perineals.
The abdominal showman
Nothing can stop the U.S. Air Corpus.
The Women's Axillary

EXAMPLES:
He was given a Bavarian enema.

Raymond Henkin, MD, Bloomfield Hills, MI

The square of the hypothalamus equals . . .

Marvin G. Gregory, MD, Nashville, TN

"The Girl from Treponema"

Louia DiBacco, D.O., Aldan, PA

The Incredible Gurney

Malcolm Phillips, MD, Great Neck, NY

Intransigent scheming attack

Sylvia Bernstein, Far Rockaway, NY

A neonate with ambitious genitalia

Thomas J. Durkin, Jr., MD, Fort Washington, PA

Iconoclastic dwarfism

Richard J. Gimpelson, MD, Chesterfield, MO

Paroxysmal nocturnal dipsomania

Sandra W. Moss, MD, Metuchen, NJ

The Charcoal joint of late syphilis

Donald Barkan, MD, Swampscott, MA

Self-assured, he answered omphalically.

Joseph A. Troncale, MD, New Holland, PA

The inflammation superhighway

Joseph B. Szgalsky, MD, Woodbury, NJ

The Seminole vesicles

Charles W. Webb, MD, Owosso, MI

"Angels prostate fall."

Dr. and Mrs. Thomas K. Rosvanis, Trafford, PA

A patient with promiscuous anemia

Burnell D. Stripling, MD, Marinette, WI

Non compos meatus

Dan W. Chiles, MD, Placentia, CA

The contraptions were five minutes apart.

Patrick M. Boccagno, MD, Altoona, PA

Polyps of the cologne

Frank P. Reynolds, MD, Jacksonville, FL

Protecting widows and endorphins

Jonathan S. Ehrlich, MD, Atlanta, GA

Sentenced to a penile colony

James A. Canfield, MD, New York, NY

A game of Tibial Pursuit

Bernard Smyle, MD, Ventura, CA

Patients with uncontrolled diabetes are subject to urinary confections.

Donald Barkan, MD, Swampscott, MA

Since he read *The Taming of the Sprue,* he's no longer a gluten for punishment.

Ivan M. Safonoff, MD, New York, NY

Worried about a mad dog bite? Get some rabbi's shots in the abdomen.

Dr. and Mrs. Michael G. Pierik, West Kingston, RI

The infectious disease staff fornicated the OR with a spray bomb.

Morris Spielberg, MD, Brooklyn, NY

The patient with PID was treated with a course of wide-speculum antibiotics.

Harry D. Cohen, MD, Oxnard, CA

A fibroid eucharist.

Frank Bruno, MD, Columbia, MD

ON THE RACK

ASSIGNMENT:
Since many magazines are weighted with medical articles, it is a matter of time until these periodicals change their names to reflect this focus. Devise such titles, plus subjects.

EXAMPLES:
Papular Mechanics—dermatologic maneuvers
Gnashional Geognathics—orthodontics
Torts Illustrated—juicy malpractice cases

EXAMPLES:
Med Magazine—"What, me worry about health care?"
Brendan O. Duterte, MD, San Jose, CA

Newswok—For sufferers of Chinese restaurant syndrome
Carl M. Pesta, DO, Warren, MI

Non Appetit—The anorexics' monthly
Jerome W. Lehrfeld, MD, Levittown, NY

Condo Nasty—World resorts that have failed health inspections
Russell J. Cox, Gastonia, NC

Emit—A news magazine for dyslexics
Stephen L. Kaufman, MD, San Francisco, CA

Herper's Bizarre—The wacky world of fever blisters
Jonathan S. Ehrlich, MD, Atlanta, GA

Better Homes and Gardenella—Infections around the house
Douglas R. Eisenstein, DO, Tucson, AZ

Psychle World—Motorbikers' maladjustments
Rev. Paul C. Hewett, Chicago, IL

Sanity Fair—Psychoneurotics' correspondence medium
Meyer C. Hodes, MD, East Rockaway, NY

Food and Whine—The psychological manifestations of eating disorders
Ethan Flaks, MD, East Syracuse, NY

Pharm Journal—What's new in drug therapy
Doris E. Fletcher, Kendall Park, NJ

TB Guide—Mycobacterial journeys
Irving Thorne, MD, Minneapolis, MN

Ladies Heme Journal—Anemia stories
Susan S. Auffiger, MD, Jamesville, NY

Oui—Easy reads in urology
Pamela Chappen, Danville, PA

Yawn Appetit—Sleep and eating disorders
Edgar A. Carvelo, MD, Napa, CA

CNS News and Whirled Report—For the latest in vertigo
Mike Kelly, MD, Buffalo, IA

Wait Watchers—How to charge MDs for overbooking their appointments
Philip Paul, MD, Miami, FL

MEDICINE BALL

ASSIGNMENT:
During the baseball strike, how could health care workers help out on the field?

EXAMPLES:
Malpractice attorney—Familiar with foul territory
Physiotherapist—Expert in seventh-inning stretches
Psychiatrist—Plays left field like a pro
Pathologist—Rules on the final out

EXAMPLES:
Orthopedist—Nails the plate with his hard-breaking stuff
Ivan M. Safonoff, MD, New York, NY

Cardiologist—Good feeling for the baseline; sends murmurs through the crowd.
Burnell D. Stripling, MD, Marinette, WI

Gastroenterologist—Reliever who comes in to prevent more runs
James J. Smith, MD, Tempe, AZ; Neil D. Wallen, MD, Bristol, TN

Pediatric urologist—Likes to perform the hidden ball trick
Melvin J. Breite, MD, Bayside, NY.

Neurosurgeon—Clears the upper deck
Brendan O. Duterte, MD, San Jose, CA

Family practitioner—Covers all the bases
Keith Guinn, MD, Butler, AL

Craniotomist—Has a wicked splitter
Joseph F. J. Curi, Torrington, CT

Respiratory therapist—Can blow it by them

W. E. Watkins, MD, Nampa, ID

Drs. DeBakey and Cooley—Texas Leaguers

Stephen L. Lieberman, MD, Clackamas, OR

Drug company rep—Relief pitcher

Robert H. Frankenfeld, MD, Long Beach, CA

Public health nurse—Makes multiple home runs

Carl Sorgen, MD, Poughkeepsie, NY

Audiologist—Good judge of pitch

S. Jay Hirsh, MD, Chester, PA

Substance abuse specialist—Catches high poppers

Rita M. Quero, MD, Ft. Myers, FL

Coroner—Makes all the tags

David A. Kline, MD, Los Angeles, CA

Circumciser—Good cutoff man

Arthur N. Feinberg, MD, Kalamazoo, MI

Physiatrist—Delivers the intentional walk

Douglas Ackerman, MD, Clackamas, OR

Barnaby Starr, MD, Baltimore, MD

Laryngologist—Expert in low and high pitches

Grafton C. Fanney, Jr., MD, Euclid, OH

OB—Catches both ends of a double-header

Michael G. Pierik, MD, W. Kingston, RI

Occupational therapist—Executes squeeze play

Louis DiBacco, DO, Aldan, PA

Dr. Kevorkian—Master of suicide squeeze
                         J. F. Gardner, MD, San Antonio, TX

Psychiatrist—Deals with all types of screwballs
                         Kieran G. Kammerer, MD, Hallowell, ME

Oncologist—Pitcher opposing the mets
                         Mark Eller, MD, Rockville, MD

AGONISTS AND PROTAGONISTS

ASSIGNMENT:
Alter the names of characters seen in nonmedical reading to qualify for their entry in the medical sphere.

EXAMPLES:
Calp-hurnia—Caesar's trussworthy wife

Sam Spadias—Urological investigator

Julius Scissor—Nonscalpel surgeon general

Madame Ovary—Gynecologist, emma-tic user

Sir Lance-a-lot—Experienced abscess-pricker with a round surgical table

ENTRIES:
Been Her—Successfully sex-changed charioteer
> Michael McNamara, MD, High Point, NC

Pokaholinus—Native American phlebotomist
> Van D. Stone, MD, Tupelo, MS

Sphincterton—Madama Butterfly's incontinence surgeon
> Douglas Ackerman, MD, Clackamas, OR

Yocesarean—Kafkaesque OB (having been through Heller), prohibited from incisional deliveries until after baby is born
> Robert H. Frankenfeld, MD, Long Beach, CA

Sure-lock Holmes—Rest-home franchisee with all patients restrained
> William F. Broeckel, MD, Yreka, CA

Cystadeno de Bergerac—Would-be OB-GYN whose nose kept getting in the way, eventually became a pathologist
> Jerome W. Lehrfeld, MD, Levittown, NY

Coldfinger—Raynaud's-afflicted evil nemesis of James Bond
> Gregory L. Smith, MD, Indianapolis, IN

Old Kinked Colon—GI endoscopist: he called for his pipe, he called for his bowel . . .

Doris E. Fletcher, Kendall Park, NJ

Rigorlento—Medical examiner notoriously slow in arriving at homicide scene

Donald Barkan, MD, Swampscott, MA

Healthcliff—Tortured English doctor who finds true love while ministering to Yorkshire's poor

Arthur LaMontagne, MD, Manchester, CT

Hem-Ophelia—Yet another inherited burden for Hamlet

Ivan M. Safonoff, MD, New York, NY

Hannibal Vector—Insatiable cardiologist

Joseph F. J. Curi, MD, Torrington, CT

Fu Man Toux—Chinese TB pulmonologist

Louis DiBacco, DO, Aldan, PA

Don Gynovanni—Overamorous woman specialist

Bruce J. Ebbels, MD, Watertown, NY

Roentgen-Tin-Tin—Veterinary radiologist

Luann Woods, DO, Ada, OK

Anti-Maim—Led campaign vs. surgical malpractice

Richard H. Morris, MD, Harrison, OH

Lady Lackbreath—Pneumothorax mistress

Melvin J. Breite, MD, Bayside, NY

THE SHORES OF TIPPLE-Y

ASSIGNMENT:
Concoct names of watering holes owned by medical entrepreneurs.

EXAMPLES:
The Waterman's Pen—Urologist
Spiritus Integumenti—Dermatologist
The Catcher in the Rye—Obstetrician

ENTRIES:
City Lytes—Nephrologist

Russell J. Cox, MD, Gastonia, NC

The Hole in the Wall—Laparoscopist

A. E. Mgebroff, MD, Yoakum, TX

Polly's Dipsia—Endocrinologist

Floyd T. Nasuti, MD, Philadelphia, PA

The Patella Tap Room—Neurologist

Meyer B. Hodes, MD, Oceanside, NY

Epstein Bar—Infections disease specialist

Robert M. Pickoff, MD, Somerset, NJ

Langerhans's Lagerhaus—Diabetologist

Doris E. Fletcher, Kendall Park, NJ

The Orchid Crypt—Pediatric urologist

Douglas Ackerman, MD, Clackamas, OR

The Plastered Joint—Orthopedist

Edward M. Sessa, MD, Schenectady, NY

Tavernus Hemangioma—Dermatologist

Mark Wiedemann, MD, Saginaw, MI

The I Surge Inn—Ophthalmologist

Douglas R. Eisenstein, DO, Tucson, AZ

The Rhine Wine Cellar—Otolaryngologist

Keith O. Wilson, MD, Norman, OK

The Bent Elbow—Orthopedist

J. J. Scarano, MD, Bradenton, FL

Ticker Doctor's Liquor Locker—Cardiologist

Melvin J. Breite, MD, Bayside, NY

The Oeno File—Toxicologist

Donald Barkan, MD, Swampscott, MA

The Pump Room—Cardiologist

Ralph M. Kniseley, MD, Oak Ridge, TN

The Whooping Trough—Pediatrician

Alan L. Goldman, MD, Raleigh, NC

The Pinta Ail—Infectious disease specialist

J. Douglas Pinney, MD, Ruxton, MD

Cuckoo's Nest—Psychiatrist

Arthur LaMontagne, MD, Manchester, CT

The Out Back—Chiropractors

M. R. Holman, MD, Amory, MS

Speak Easy—Pulmonologist

Morey Filler, MD, San Francisco, CA

The Rusty Zipper—Incontinence specialists

Joseph B. Szgalsky, MD, Woodbury, NJ

Lithotipsy's—Urologist

Sherrell L. Beecher, Rancho Santa Fe, CA

The Spinal Tap—Neurologist

Richard H. Morris, MD, Harrison, OH

Charcot's Joint—Syphilologist

Fred Freeman, MD, Manhattan, KS

Bottoms Up—Proctologist

W. E. Watkins, MD, Nampa, ID

Gyn and Tonic (contractions) Inn—OB

Louis DiBacco, MD, Aldan, PA

The Bottom Line—Hospital administrator

M. David Lauter, MD, York, ME

The Bleary Eye—Ophthalmologist

Raymond Bechtle, Minnetonka, MN

In Vino Veritas—Harvard grads, regardless of specialty

Anatoly Belilovsky, MD, Brooklyn, NY

GREAT WORDS

ASSIGNMENT:
Fit a great saying to answer a question in the medical sphere.

EXAMPLES:
What is good advice for a resident in a pyramid program?
"Don't look back. Something may be gaining on you."

The plaintiff will call off the malpractice suit for a token settlement
What say?
"Millions for defense, but not one cent for tribute."

Realistically, what can you advise diabetics bent on a day of binge
eating?
"Let them eat cake."

How did you fare in the herpes simplex epidemic?
"Read my lips."

What is your impression of the direction of health care?
"A riddle wrapped in a mystery inside an enigma."

ENTRIES:
What does the chief resident say to the new crop of interns?
"Who's on first?"

Meyer B. Hodes, MD, East Rockaway, NY

What's the end point for liposuction?
"It's not over till the fat lady sings."

Ivan M. Safonoff, MD, New York, NY

What is a hedging radiologist's X-ray interpretation philosophy?
"When you come to a fork in the road, take it."

Joseph F. J. Curi, MD, Torrington, CT

What is your response to the charge of unoriginal work in your journal article?
"When you steal from one author, it's plagiarism; if you steal from many, it's research."

Donald Barkan, MD, Swampscott, MA

Irate orthopedist to resident: What do you mean there's no fiberglass left?
"We'll always have Paris."

Louis DiBacco, MD, Aldan, PA

Will catheterization bear results?
"Aprés moi le déluge."

Stephen L. Kaufman, MD, San Francisco, CA
Jonathan S. Ehrlich, MD, Atlanta, GA

What was the hospital administrator's plea to the fractious medical staff?
"Why can't we all just get along?"

Robert A. Howard, MD, Bryan, TX

What did the Shakespearean bariatrician supplicate?
"O! that this too, too solid flesh should melt, thaw and resolve itself
   into a dew."

Jerome W. Lehrfeld, MD, Levittown, NY

Why wouldn't you donate or receive a renal transplant?
"Neither a borrower nor a lender be."

Morey Filler, MD, San Francisco, CA

What comfort can the urologist give to one with a low ureteral stone?
"This, too, shall pass . . ."

Douglas R. Eisenstein, DO, Tucson, AZ

MEMOIRS

ASSIGNMENT:
Compose a fitting title for the summary of one's iatric career.

EXAMPLES:
Forty Years Under the Lash—Ophthalmologist
The Long Gray Line—Geriatrics
The Catcher in the Rye—Alcoholic obstetrician
My Compressed Story—Physiotherapist
Confessions of a Radicle Conservative—Neurologist

ENTRIES:
The Canker-Beriberi Tales—Tropical disease expert
Meyer B. Hodes, MD, East Rockaway, NY

The Prince and the Pauper—Neurosurgeon-turned-pediatrician
Grafton C. Fanney, MD, Euclid, OH

A Separate Piece—Trauma surgeon
Robert Allison, MD, Panorama City, CA

Count Scapula—Orthopedist who moonlit as a phlebotomist
Barni Schlein, Richmond, VA

By the Skin of Our Teeth—Teratoma expert
Steve Lieberman, MD, Clackamas, OR

Jane Eyre—Anonymous female ENT
Irving Thorne, MD, Minneapolis, MN

Tales from the CryptOrchid—Pediatric urologist
Douglas Ackerman, MD, Clackamas, OR

Eye the Jury—Forensic ophthalmologist
Joseph F. J. Curi, MD, Torrington, CA

The pHiladelphia Story—Metabolist, acid-based along the Mainline
Doris E. Fletcher, Kendall Park, NJ

Remembrance of Things Passed—Urologist
Neil DeNunzio, MD, Winfall, NC

The Wizard of Os—Gynecologist
Edward M. Thompson, MD, Mechanicsburg, PA

The Idiot—Rural, independent, fee-for-service MD
Ted McMahon, MD, Seattle, WA

Gone With the Mind—Psychiatrist
Morey Filler, MD, San Francisco, CA

The Memoirs of Castanova—Amorous orthopedist
Ivan M. Safonoff, MD, New York, NY

Legend of the Falls—The best geriatric orthopedist in the country
Russell J. Cox, MD, Gastonia, NC

A Long Day's Journey into Night—Anesthesiologist
Malcolm C. Phillips, MD, Bronx, NY

CLINICAL TRIAL

ASSIGNMENT:
Superimpose medical lingo upon legal in a court of law.

EXAMPLES:
"I rest my case," unburdened the surgical supply salesman.
"I'll see you in chambers." blinked the ophthalmologist.
"May I approach the bench?" asked the surgeon of long-standing.
"Habeas corpus," embodied the pathologist.

ENTRIES:
"I object," declared the ER doc, finding a foreign body through the ophthalmoscope."

Steve Lieberman, MD, Clackamas, OR

"Order, order in the court," beseeched the obsessive-compulsive psychiatrist.
"Two cheeseburgers," requested the perennially starving intern.

Morey Filler, MD, San Francisco, CA

"I have a warrant for your arrest," charged the cardiologist.

Karen L. Mutter, DO, and Lynne Walder, Tampa, FL

"You are going to do hard time," the lithotripser was told.

Burnell Stripling, MD, Marinette, WI

"I hereby sentence you to hard labor in solitary confinement," said the obstetrician.

Ralph M. Kniseley, MD, Oak Ridge, TN

"Due to an assault with a cutlass, the deceased was declared intestate."

Raymond E. Joseph, MD, Philadelphia, PA

"Have you reached a decision?" questioned the intern of the pathologist.

Eugene Cullen, MD, Harrisburg, PA

"Ladies and gentlemen of the jury," thundered the peer reviewer.

Gary M. Gorlick, MD, Los Angeles, CA

"My client has been framed," said the optometrist.

Melvin J. Breite, MD, Bayside, NY

"When do I take the stand?" asked the scrub nurse.

Donald Barkan, MD, Swampscott, MA

"May I have the judge's ear?" whispered the audiologist.

Joel T. Appleton, MD, Abilene, TX

"Hear ye, hear ye," drummed the otologist.

Arthur E. LaMontagne, MD, Manchester, CT

"Your Honor," said one physician to the other on the 18th tee.

Douglas Ackerman, MD, Clackamas, OR

"Raise your right hand," directed the motion-range-checking physiatrist.

Lourdes Romano-Jana, MD, Erie, PA

UNDESIDERATA

ASSIGNMENT:
Create a medical equivalent to needing something like a hole in the head.

EXAMPLES:
He/she needs/needed that like . . .

. . . an ophthalmologist needs a tremor.

. . . a radiologist needs diplopia.

. . . a neurosurgeon needs generalized pruritus.

. . . Don Giovanni needed Peyronie's disease.

. . . Joe Montana needed Dupuytren's contracture.

ENTRIES

. . . a principal ballet dancer needs a hydrocele.

Thuan L. Tran, MD, Claremont, CA

. . . Captain Hook needed pruritus ani.

Joseph A. Troncale, MD, New Holland, PA

. . . a sleep lab needs an espresso machine.

Douglas Ackerman, MD, Clackamas, OR

. . . a dowser needs water on the knee.

Joel T. Appleton, MD, Abilene, TX

. . . Wynton Marsalis needs oral herpes simplex.

Susan L. Auffinger, MD, Jamesville, NY

. . . a CPR rescuer needs a sneezing fit.

Brendan O. Duterte, MD, San Jose, CA

. . . an obstetrician needs a night job.

Morey Filler, MD, San Francisco, CA

. . . a poison control volunteer needs dyslexia.

Alan L. Goldman, MD, Raleigh, NC

. . . an orthopedist needs fine leather gloves.

Richard A. Weddle, MD, Bloomington, IN

. . . a sumo wrestler needs anorexia.

Michael Levin, MD, San Ramon, CA

. . . A Parkinsonian needs an earthquake while trying to eat peas.

E. M. Herrera, MD, Lincoln Park, MI

. . . A hypochondriac needs a job in the ICU.

Sandra Mamis, RPA-C, Poughkeepsie, NY

. . . an anorexic needs a tapeworm.

James R. Logan, MD, Paradise, CA

. . . a pediatrician's reception room needs a set of drums.

Ralph C. Merwin, DO, Harrison, AR

. . . the Tin Man needs ambulatory cardiac monitoring.

Doris E. Fletcher, Kendall Park, NJ

. . . a man with priapism needs to read *Penthouse* magazine.

Steve Lieberman, MD, Clackamas, OR

. . . a junior medical student needs to third-assist on a laparoscopic inguinal hernia repair.

Allen Solum, MD, Paynesville, MN

. . . a dentist needs hiccups (on either side of the chair).

Sylvia Bernstein, Far Rockaway, NY

. . . a proctologist needs hyperosmia.

Ivan Safonoff, MD, NYC
Stan Hines, MD, Huntsville, TX
Mark Wiedemann, MD, Saginaw, MI

IN THE SWING

ASSIGNMENT:
Apply golf terms to medical situations.

EXAMPLES:
Hole in one—Lumbar puncture on the first try
Pebble Beach—The lithotripsy suite
Match play—That which perpetuates the burn service
Wind shot—Injection to relieve asthma
Scratch player—A dermatologist

ENTRIES:
Fore-skins—Golf game played by urologists for money
Arthur E. LaMontagne, Jr., MD, Manchester, CT

On the senior tour—Nursing home physician
Douglas Ackerman, MD, Clackamas, OR

Grant relief—Return a benign diagnosis
Robert G. Satterfield, MD, Hermitage, TN

Back nine—Medium-sized chiropractic group
Ted McMahon, MD, Seattle, WA

Flop shot—B-12 for anything but a B-12 deficiency
Willis L. Dixon, MD, East Grand Rapids, MI

The greens—First-year residents
Richard D. Otto, MD, North Bend, OR

Pin high—Directions from mammoplasty patient
William M. Oppenheimer, MD, Richmond, VA

Water hazard—"Okay, now bear down."
James A. Krug, MD, Olympia, WA

Mulligan—Another attempt at phlebotomy

> David Fall, MD, Gilette, WY

Pot bunker—Liposuction candidate

> Joseph Grayzel, MD, Englewood, NJ

Hook shot—Tetanus booster for clumsy fishermen

> Paul A. Roozeboom, MD, Racine, WI

Shotgun start—Prelude to trauma unit nightmare

> William Kellett, MD, Greenville, SC

Stroke and distance—Transfer of CVA patient to faraway tertiary care center

> David P. Schneider, MD, Bedford, IN

Caddy—What the doctor used to drive before he got the Benz

> Melvin J. Breite, MD, Bayside, NY

Improving one's lie—Continuously adding to nonexistent credentials

> Meyer B. Hodes, MD, Oceanside, NY

Slow play—The hypothyroid invitational

> Stephen Lieberman, MD, Clackamas, OR

Public links course—An epidemiologist at work

> I. J. Friedman, MD, Washington, MO

Miller Barber and Lee Trephino—Early brain surgeons

> Joel D. Lilly, MD, Seattle, WA

Approach iron—Advice to hematologist with anemic patient

> Joel T. Appleton, Abilene, TX

Driving range—Distance between specialist's country club and hospital

> Bob Martino, MD, Sundance, WY

...BUT NO CIGAR

ASSIGNMENT:

In the same vein as 6-Up, Victoria's Partial Disclosure, the Macroscope, and Platinumfinger, contrive a medical near-miss which, if foreseen, would have made all the difference.

EXAMPLES:

Billroth 0.5   Extensor digiti sexti   The Milligram stain
Vitreous wit   Carpal ditch

ENTRIES:

Light Obfuscation by Stimulated Emission of Radiation (LOSER)
>   Jonathan S. Ehrlich, MD, Atlanta GA

Creek of Schlemm
>   Charles W. Webb, MD, Corunna, MI

Hemisemidemitendinosis
>   Paul J. Nuccio, MD, Tacoma, WA

American Medical Club
>   Glenn H. Perelson, MD, Bonita, CA

Addisonian predicament
>   Sandra Mamis PA-C, Poughkeepsie, NY

Institutionalized hernia
>   David M. Pease, MD, Estill, SC

Mons mercurialis
>   David Barkan, MD, Swampscott, MA

Straw fever
>   S.D. Madduri, MD, Poplar Bluff, MO

Crawl space membrane
>   Marc S. Williams, MD, La Crosse, WI

Zebracampus

Daniel Schual-Berke, MD, Seattle, WA

Cryptdaisyism

E. Gallenstein, MD, Cincinnati, OH

Cribriform saucer

Meyer B. Hodes, MD, East Rockaway, NY

Employee aureus

Steven Preston, MD, Harrisburg, PA

Eleventorium

Hugh H. Wang, MD, Clayton, CA

Cushing's suspicion

Ivan M. Safonoff, MD, New York, NY

Half astrocytomna

Timothy R. Hopf, MD, Denver, CO

Brutusean section

Morey Filler, MD, San Francisco, CA

Gillette test (for diphtheria)

H. Peter Barnes, MD, South Yarmouth, MA

Medial latitudinal fasciculus

Richard A. Mingione, MD, Atlantic City, NJ

Charcot's disreputable gathering place

Joseph F. J. Curi, MD, Torrington, CT

Rest stop au lait spots

Robert R. Jones, MD, Nevada, MO

Extracorporeal shock ripple lithotripsy

Stephen Lieberman, MD, Clackamas, OR

Gleno-serious dislocation

Allan B. Solum, MD, Paynesville, MN

The bronchial bush

Neal Green, MD, Corsicana, TX

The H-III virus

Marcus Miller, MD, Sidney, OH

Bowman's tablet

Douglas Ackerman, MD, Clackamas, OR

Blackian movement

Daniel P. Sporn, MD, Athens, PA

The Mamanicolaou smear

Julio Novoa, MD, Lutherville, MD

Hippoplasty

Mark A. Samia, MD, Raleigh, NC

Subcontinents of Langerhans

Christopher W. Groner, MD, Jonesville, NC

PATHO-FINDER

ASSIGNMENT:
Invent a disease.

EXAMPLES:
Berpes—long virally-induced, seed-catalog-vectored periods of silence, punctuated by eruptions or eructations

Spumonia—Lung lesions caused by excessive ingestion of Italian ice cream

Mani-Years' disease—A cluster of geriatric conditions

Turret's syndrome—Vestibular deficit caused by too much association with naval artillery

The Frescabaldi defect—Hair loss associated with soft drink excesses

ENTRIES:
Status arithmeticus—Inability to progress to algebra and geometry from simple arithmetic

Tejinder S. Sandhu, MD, Sanger, CA

Mnemonia—Overuse of memory devices, prevalent in medical students

Arthur N. Feinberg, MD, Kalamazoo, MI

Picknickian syndrome—Compulsion to eat alfresco

Joseph J. Scarano, MD, Bradenton, FL

Schusstosomiasis—A flukey dysentery that strikes on ski slopes

Doris E. Fletcher, Kendall Park, NJ

Snappledema—Orbital bloating caused by overindulgence in iced tea

Joseph F. J. Curi, MD, Torrington, CT

Oculobrachioradialis crisis—Simultaneous spasm of extraocular and forearm pronator muscles from frequent glances at wristwatch during long lectures

Robert C. Whitesitt, MD, Helena, MT

Münchausen's syndrome—Total depletion of provisions from fake appetite

Scott Treatman, DO, Cazenovia, NY

Discardia—Gin rummy players' palpitations caused by worry over throwing away the wrong card

Alan L. Goldman, MD, Raleigh, NC

Gatekeeper's thumb—Painful thumb inflammation from excessive authorization referral forms

Timothy R. Hopf, MD, Denver, CO

Scarlett fever—Compulsive problem deferment (till tomorrow) because others, frankly, don't give a damn

Sylvia Bernstein, Far Rockaway, NY

Neiman-Pick disease—Degenerative disorder associated with expensive department store shopping

Joel T. Appleton, MD, Abilene, TX

Add-a-son's disease—Inability to bear female offspring

Martin S. Lipton, MD, Carmel, NY

Wickets—Bowleg condition invariably associated with mallet finger

Robert R. Jones, MD, Nevada, MO

Condominium accuminatum—Acquisition affliction of the all-too-wealthy

Douglas Ackerman, MD, Clackamas, OR

Alopizza—Patchy hair loss caused by noxious fumes in Italian kitchens

Arthur E. LaMontagne, Jr., MD, Manchester, CT

Lithotipsy—Consequences of drinking too much from a stone beer mug

Neal Green, MD, Corsicana, TX

Guidlinitis drastica—A syndrome of rigidity, tremulousness, and torpor

Meyer B. Hodes, MD, East Rockaway, NY

Staff infection—Shepherd's disease: erythema and swelling of the hand that holds the crook

Gene Westveer, MD, Zeeland, MI

Dysparheumia—Postcoital aching of every single joint and muscle in your body after age sixty.

Julio Novoa, MD, Lutherville, MD

Leukopenia—Pallor of the phallus

E. Gallenstein, MD, Cincinnati, OH

Toxic sock syndrome—Febrile illness associated with excessive use of superabsorbent hose

Ronald P. Olah, MD, Pasadena, CA

TAX-I-TERMIST

ASSIGNMENT:
If the IRS were to send an agent to personally collect your taxes, conceive words of greeting for him/her.

EXAMPLES:
"Ah, a fellow seizure specialist!"—Neurologist
"I've heard of oxygen debt, but this is ridiculous!"—Physiologist
" 'Sblood, thou stinkard."—Shakespearean hematologist
"I thought I'd seen all the day's morbidity up to now."—Pathologist

ENTRIES:
"You do the pushing and you expect me to deliver?"—Obstetrician

Julio Novoa, MD, Lutherville, MD

"Do you believe in professional courtesy?"—Proctologist

Douglas Ackerman, MD, Clackamas, OR

"You can have everything I collect today."—Parasitologist

Melvin J. Breite, MD, Bayside, NY

"I'd love to visit with you, but we're under cholera quarantine."—Infectious disease specialist

Morey Filler, MD, San Francisco, CA

"I can take care of those ears, but later you will need to see a good dentist."—Plastic surgeon

Tejinder S. Sandhu, MD, Sanger, CA

"The math may be a little off. I only know how to count backward from one hundred."—Anesthesiologist

Kathy Waller, MD, Fort Collins, CO

"I see you majored in collectivization."—Medical school dean of admissions

Joel T. Appleton, MD, Abilene, TX

"I hear you knocking, but you can't come in."—Audiologist

Ritchie C. Shoemaker, MD, Pocomoke City, MD

"I feel as if more than my sinuses are draining."—Allergist

Neal Green, MD, Corsicana, TX

"Be with you in a minute. Have a stool."—Gastroenterologist

Mackenzie Smith, MD, Mercer Island, WA

"Uh-huh. Ummm. I see . . . I'll give you one hour."—Psychiatrist

Edward M. Thompson, MD, Mechanicsburg, PA.

"I'm exempt. I'm ataxic."—Neurologist

Scott Treatman, DO, Cazenovia, NY

"You've come to take my pound of flesh."—Dermatologist

Floyd T. Nasuti, MD, Philadelphia, PA

"Come to twist my arm?"—Physiatrist

Meyer B. Hodes, MD, Oceanside, NY

"Ah yes, I've been expecting you. My life is full of excisions."—Surgeon

Charles G. Eschenburg, MD, Delray Beach, FL

THE GREAT BREAKTHROUGH

ASSIGNMENT:
Compose a title for a scientific paper that describes the conquest of a specific disease.

EXAMPLES:
"Cluster's Last Stand"—Headache
"The Conquered Grape"—Alcoholism
"The Ecstasy of Defeat"—Bunions
"Just in the Nicotine"—Tobacco addiction

ENTRIES:
"VD Vici"—STDs

Daniel K. Jass, MD, Lawrenceville, NJ

"The Clot Thickens"—Hemophilia

Alan L. Goldman, MD, Raleigh, NC

"Tse, Tse, Tsetse Good-bye"—African sleeping sickness

Stephen L. Kaufman, MD, San Francisco, CA

"Clung Lung Sprung"—Pulmonary fibrosis

Charles G. Eschenburg, MD, Delray Beach, FL

"Moon Struck"—Cushing's disease

Leonard Schreier, MD, Bloomfield Hills, MI

"Beriberi Buried"—Vitamin B deficiency

Tejinder S. Sandhu, MD, Sanger, CA

"And the Beat Goes On"—Third-degree heart block

Joseph B. Segalsky, MD, Woodbury, NJ

"Nipped in the Bud"—Stoma elimination

Rajenda K. Arora, MD, Orange, NJ

"The Taming of the Hue"—Jaundice

Edward M. Thompson, MD, Mechanicsburg, PA

"Last Tangle in Parous"—Umbilical cord complications

Neal Green, MD, Corsicana, TX

"To Kill a Mockingbird"—Echolalia

Steven Preston, MD, Harrisburg, PA

"Watership Down"—Priapism

Charles W. Webb, MD, Corunna, MI

"Cankers Away"—Aphthous stomatitis

Doris E. Fletcher, MD, Kendall Park, NJ

"Thanks for the Memory"—Alzheimer's disease

David G. Covell, MD, Pasadena, CA

"All Quiet on the Intestinal Front"—Borborygmi

Robert O. Frank, MD, Norwich, NY

"A Trichy Solution"—Specific STD

Morey Filler, MD, San Francisco, CA

"Kiss Your RAST Good-bye"—Allergies

Stanley S. Paras, MD, Bedford, NH

"The Final Four"—Erythema Infectiosum (5th Disease)

Kathy Waller, MD, Fort Collins, CO

"Memory Loss? Forget It"—Alzheimer's disease

Melvin J. Breite, MD, Bayside, NY

"The Thrill Is Over"—Aortic stenosis

Charles W. Webb, MD, Corunna, MI

"The Welt Is Our Oyster"—Hives

Ted McMahon, MD, Seattle, WA

"Extra Xtra: Read All about It"—Turner's syndrome
Eugene Cullen, MD, Harrisburg, PA

"The Blast Is in the Past"—Leukemia
Russell J. Cox, MD, Gastonia, NC

"The Pleasure of His Company"—Dyspareunia
Joel T. Appleton, MD, Abilene, TX

"Serum: No de Bergerac"—Rhinoplasty produced by an injectable immunotherapy
Robert D. Lafsky, MD, Reston, VA

"Do You Know the Way to Sans Toupee?"—Male pattern baldness
Thomas J. Durkin, Jr., MD, Fort Washington, PA

REFUND REQUESTED

ASSIGNMENT:
Describe the misunderstanding that brought a medical person to the box office to complain.

EXAMPLES:
The physical therapist expected to hear Beethoven's *Postural* Symphony.
The infectious disease specialist expected *Six Degrees of Suppuration*.
The orthopedist—*The Odd Carpal*.
The ophthalmologist—Bram Stoker's *Macula*.
The podiatrist—*Joan of Arch*.

ENTRIES:
Managed-care executive—*Raiders of the Lost Art*.
David A. Kline, MD, Los Angeles, CA

Sonographer—*The Picture of Dorrie in Gray*.
Julio Novoa, MD, Lutherville, MD

Interventional cardiologist—*A Midsummer Night's Ream*.
Hugh H. Wang, MD, Concord, CA

HMO medical director—*The Threepenny Operrati*.
Anatoly Belilovsky, MD, Brooklyn, NY

Urologist—*Detrusor Consequences*.
David A. Zornick, MD, Bristol, CT

Endocrinologist—*On Her Majesty's Secreting Service*.
David M. Pease, MD, Estill, SC

Dentist—*Glencaries, Glenn Floss*.
Alison Maggio, RN, Islip, NY

Geneticist—*Helix the Cat*.
Doris E. Fletcher, Kendall Park, NJ

Cardiologist—*Stent of a Woman.*

Matthew J. Burday, DO, Wilmington, DE

Pulmonologist—*The Empyema Strikes Back.*

Thuan L. Tran, MD, Claremont, CA

Urologist—*Epididymis Rex.*

Arthur E. LaMontagne, Jr., MD, Manchester, CT

Nutritionist—*Madame Butterfat.*

Melvin J. Breite, MD, Bayside, NY

Nephrologist—*Loop Dreams.*

Joseph A. Trancale, MD, New Holland, PA

ICD9 coder—*Kubric's 200.1.*

Jonathan S. Ehrlich, MD, Atlanta, GA

Endocrinologist—*The Silence of the Glands.*

Roger Goldberg, Pensacola, FL

Urologist—*Two Gentlemen of Peyronie.*

Thomas J. Durkin, MD, Washington, PA

Dermatologist—*A Pox on Lips Now.*

B. J. Cochrane, MD, Watertown, WI

Bariatrician—*The Count of Monte Crisco.*

Joel T. Appleton, MD, Abilene, TX

Public health physician—*The Enigma Vaccinations.*

Brant Tedrow, MD, Groveport, OH

Podiatrist—*Raisers of the Lost Arch.*

Michael W. Swanson, MD, Greenfield, MA

Speech pathologist—*Schindler's Lisp.*

Joseph F. J. Curi, MD, Torrington, CT

Speech pathologist—*Stuttering Heights*.

Patrick M. Boccagno, MD, Altoona, PA

Sex-change surgeon—*Been Her*.

Albert T. Gros, MD, Austin, TX

Gynecologist—*The Wizard of Os*.

Joanne Liegner, MD, Newton, NJ

Sex therapist—*Beethoven's Erotica Symphony*.

Arthur N. Feinberg, MD, Kalamazoo, MI

Neurologist—*Leaving Las Vagus*.

Sidney G. Piness, MD, Plainfield, NJ

HARMONIC MONICKERS

ASSIGNMENT:
Fancifully name the progeny of the well-known to yield medical terminology.

EXAMPLES:
Dan Blocker—Beta   John Keats—Spiro
Gary Hart—Phoetyl   Cristóbal Colón—Sigmoid

ENTRIES:
Ho Chi Minh—Vita

Robert A. Fink, MD, Norfolk, VA

Johann Sebastian Bach—Hessel

Stanley Hartness, MD, Kosciusko, MS

Michael Caine—Benzo

Ronald P. Olah, MD, Pasadena, CA

Bobby Seale—Varico, Recto, Entero, and Little Sister

Stephen Lieberman, MD, Clackamas, OR

Max Factor—R. H.

Gene Westveer, MD, Zeeland, MI

Dennis Rodman—Conan

Dave Taube, Oak Harbor, WA

Marlon Brando—Generico

Melvin J. Breite, MD, Bayside, NY

Johann Sebastian Bach—Ivy Piggy

Kathy Waller, MD, Fort Collins, CO

Gabriel Heatter—Kath

Doris E. Fletcher, Kendall Park, NJ

Tommy Dorsey—Latissimus

> Alan L. Goldman, MD, Raleigh, NC

Phil Gramm—Angela Olivia (Angie O.)

> Michael J. Ichniowski, MD, Lutherville, MD

Tom Ewell—Knod

> Sylvia Bernstein, Far Rockaway, NY

Eddie Fisher—Sylvian

> Arthur N. Feinberg, MD, Kalamazoo, MI

Elihu Root—Dorsal

> Daniel J. Colombi, MD, Haddonfield, NJ

Sally Ride—Chlo

> Donald S. Brooks, MD, Redding, CA

Marge Schott—Ivy

> B. J. Cochrane, MD, Watertown, WI

Peter Lorre—Cal

> Douglas Ackerman, MD, Clackamas, OR

Patricia Neal—Perry

> Patrick M. Boccagno, MD, Altoona, PA

Guido Monalla—Sal

> Michael Dennis, MD, (no address)

Michael Foote—Claude

> Tejinder S. Sandhu, MD, Sanger, CA

SYLLABILITY

ASSIGNMENT:
Rearrange a medical term to give it an outlandish meaning. Confine it to the first syllable.

EXAMPLES:
Fystic fibrosis—Scar formation due to pugilistic career
Slammer toe—Pedal injury resulting from kicking prison bars
Floorceps—Frequently dropped surgical instrument
Dysbursitis—Agitated state due to excessive office overhead
Spreematurity—Obstetrical problem caused by excessive partying during pregnancy

ENTRIES:
Blisspareunia—The joy of sex
Joseph F. J. Curi, MD, Torrington, CT

Fadenoma—A tumor that's in the literature for just a short time
Steven Preston, MD, Harrisburg, PA

Futilization review—What they should have called this process all along
Michael J. Ichniowski, MD, Lutherville, MD

Kinfluenza—Sudden nausea, aching, and lightheadedness caused by the unexpected arrival of one's relatives
Sandra Mamis, PA-C, Poughkeepsie, NY

Fediculosis—Infestation of government agencies in medical practice
Julio Novoa, MD, Lutherville, MD

Sophthalmologist—A second-year eye resident
Barni Schlein, Richmond, VA

Heathrolithiasis—Getting stoned on a London layover between flights
Gene Westveer, MD, Zeeland, MI

Trombocytopenic purpura—Facial petechiae from forceful blowing into musical instruments

Tejinder S. Sandhu, MD, Sanger, CA

Brrrsitis—Cold-induced joint pain

Charles W. Webb, MD, Traverse City, MI

Leashmaniasis—Occupational injury seen in professional dog handlers

Russell J. Cox, MD, Gastonia, NC

Hell maintenance organization—The hereafter for all those managed-care administrators

Kathy Waller, MD, Fort Collins, CO

Clamydia—Shucker's fingers

Arthur Verdesca, MD, Morristown, NJ

Rhyme disease—Compulsion to write poetry about ticks

Joseph B. Szgalsky, MD, Woodbury, NJ

OCCUPATIONAL HAZARDS

ASSIGNMENT:
Invent injuries or illnesses related by name to the workplace or pastime where they were incurred.

EXAMPLES:
Contract dermatitis—Bridge hands' hands
Philatelectasis—Stamp collector's lung
Carnal tunnel syndrome—STD
Mixedema—Swelling peculiar to bartenders
Tic dollaroux—Nervous affliction of cashiers

ENTRIES:
Bananaphylaxis—Allergic crisis in actors who play Tarzan
Joseph F. J. Curi, MD, Torrington, CT

Belle's palsy—Endemic in the South and characterized by facial paralysis from excessive smiling during beauty pageants
Kathy Waller, MD, Fort Collins, CO

Czarcoma—Unconscious state of former Russian rulers
Daniel J. Colombi, MD, Haddonfield, NJ

Foreigngitis—Traveler's sore throat
Peggy Spencer, MD, Albuquerque, NM

Percussis—Drummer's cough
Linda LeMay, MD, and Scott Treatman, DO, Cazenovia, NY

Intersusception—Quarterback's bowel affliction
Brett Johnson, MD, Erie, PA

Appleplexy—Affliction common to orchardists and computer users
Frank P. Reynolds, MD, Jacksonville, FL

La smell indifference—Perfume worker's cold
Edward M. Thompson, MD, Dillsburg, PA

Nubergulosis—Diner's disease caused by bad lobster sauce
Joseph A. Troncale, MD, New Holland, PA

Parkingson's disease—Inherited garage attendant affliction
Stephen Petrany, MD, Huntington, NY

Condominia acumulata—Banker's foreclosure nightmare
Martin S. Lipton, MD, Carmel, NY

Pay-Saks disease—Inherited disorder characterized by compulsive shopping
Anne B. King, MD, Greensboro, NC

Car pulmonale—Heart trouble in auto-towing mechanics
Barbara Kendall, Short Hills, NJ

Granuloma linguinale—Pasta maker's nodule
Stan Hines, MD, Huntsville, TX

Friesenmonger syndrome—cardiopathy in frozen food merchants
Tejinder S. Sandhu, MD, Sanger, CA

Hexzema—Skin disorders from handling voodoo dolls
Douglas Ackerman, MD, Clackamas, OR

Wry's syndrome—Facial dystonia caused by excessive droll humor
Charles W. Webb, MD, Traverse City, MI

NEW OLD SAWS

ASSIGNMENT:
Adapt a well-known proverb to the medical world.

EXAMPLES:
A rolling stone thwarts the lithtripter.
Hyperalimentation is thicker than water.

A stitch in time can be hemostatic.
The underinsured and his money are soon parted.

ENTRIES were lost in the mail. As a substitute, these were devised by the author.

A penny saved delights the HMO.

Spare the rod and promote night vision.

Make vitamin D while the sun shines.

One swallow does not a GI series make.

It is better to have a mild STD than never to have loved at all.

Surgeons cannot live by thread alone.

Sharper than a hound's tooth is a letter from PRO

The heart has reason the EKG knows nothing of.

All that glitters is not accounts receivable.

Colonoscopists rush in where angels fear to tread.

Androgenic hormones make the man.

One good tetanus shot deserves another.

Maculae are only skin-deep.

Tonometry is in the eye of the beholder.

An ounce of laparoscopy is worth a pound of laparotomy.

The treadmill is not always to the swift.

Don't cry over spilt specimen.

Let him who is without scalpel blast the first stone.

If finger-stick is here, can phlebotomy be far behind?

Variety is the spice of family practice.

No exocrine pancreatic cell is an island.

Am I my brother's beeper?

Every X-ray film has a silver lining.

A bird in the hand risks psittacosis.

The proof of the pudding is in the antacids.

Hell hath no fury like the chief kept waiting.

Some men are born hypothyroid; some achieve hypothyroidism; some have hypothyroidism thrust upon them.

Two heads are better than one, provided they are attached to different torsos.

SPIN DOCTORS

ASSIGNMENT:

Create a spin to boost a candidate for election. Do this by using the medically routine but high-sounding.

EXAMPLES: Our candidate . . .

. . . listens to the electorate with vibrating ossicles.

. . . is homeostatic!

. . . subjects all the issues to binocular vision.

. . . will travel among the people with bipedal stride.

ENTRIES:

. . . will inspire at least twelve times a minute every day while in office.

Steven Preston, MD, Harrisburg, PA

. . . has never used an extensor tendon to flex a joint.

Grafton C. Fanney, Jr., MD, Euclid, OH

. . . can bring two sides together, help heal wounds, and take credit if it looks good.

Hugh H. Wang, MD, Concord, CA

. . . is one who possesses genuine Purkinje fiber . . . very cerebellar.

John H. Sand, MD, Ellensburg, WA

. . . has heart!

Morey Filler, MD, San Francisco, CA

. . . maintains his balance with functional proprioception.

Neil Berkowitz, MD, San Diego, CA

. . . has no osseous structural units in the closet.

Joseph F. J. Curi, MD, Torrington, CT

. . . will shake your hand with ossified phalanges.

Joseph Grayzel, MD, Englewood, NJ

. . . will osculate, without trepidation, juvenile homo sapiens.

Russell J. Cox, MD, Gastonia, NC

. . . is so kind that not even his opponents deny his sympathetic nervous system.

Alan L. Goldman, MD, Raleigh, NC

. . . has reasoning not merely tentorial, but supratentorial.

Jonathan S. Ehrlich, MD, Atlanta, GA

. . . will clean up toxic waste with biliary prowess.

Douglas Ackerman, MD, Clackamas, OR

. . . will take up your cause with beating heart.

Sanjiv Verma, MD, Oxnard, CA

. . . is stimulated by Cooper's ligament support of his constituents.

Joseph B. Szgalsky, MD, Woodbury, NJ

. . . synthesizes the issues with a symphony of synapses.

Howard Neudorf, MD, Waipahu, HI

. . . has a finger on the pulse of things, using his/her most distal phalanges.

Stan Hines, MD, Huntsville, TX

SENSE OF HUMOR

ASSIGNMENT:
Take a familiar three-word expression which has "of" in the middle. Give it a medical connotation.

EXAMPLES:
Bridge of Sighs: Device associated with tooth-loss depression
Head of Cabbage: Heart-surgery department chairman
Jack of Hearts: Defibrillator
Scales of Justice: Psoriasis in a jurist

ENTRIES:
Kiss of fire: Herpes labialis exposed to salsa verde.
W. E. Watkins, MD, Nampa, ID

Ampulla of Vater: Vot you use to mix der medicine mit
E. Gallenstein, MD, Cincinnati, OH

Jack-of-all-trades, master of none: MD, JD
Howard Wiles, MD, Richmond, VA

Reversal of fortune: Income generated by subspecialists
Steven Preston, MD, Harrisburg, PA

Clap of thunder: A severe case of gonorrhea
Meyer B. Hodes, MD, East Rockaway, NY

Stream of consciousness: Successful enuresis treatment
Sylvia Bernstein, Far Rockaway, NY

Buns of steel: Complication in aerobic, hemosiderotic dancers
Jerome Eder, MD, Agoura, CA; Joseph F. J. Curi, MD, Torrington, CT

String of pearls: Grand outpouring from attending on rounds.
Stanley Hartness, MD, Kosciusco, MS

March of Dimes: Payout from managed-care organizations
Sandra Mamis, RPA-C, Poughkeepsie, NY

One of Many: Visits to law office required to "heal" whiplash
Robert L. Hillery, MD, Findlay, OH

Labors of Hercules: Multiple birth
Karen Ilika, MD, Kirkland, WA

Chicken of the sea: Cowardly ship's doctor
D. J. Colombi, MD, Haddonfield, NJ

Stick of gum: Shot of Novocain from your dentist
Aileen Faulkner, Pittsburg, PA

Long of tooth: Older oral surgeon
Morey Filler, MD, San Francisco, CA

Pride of lions: Group of chief surgical residents
Tejiner S. Sandhu, MD, Sanger, CA

Act of faith: Yohimbine ingestion
Arthur S. Verdesca, M.D., Morristown, NJ

Tower of Babel: High-rise speech therapy clinic
Frank P. Reynolds, MD, Jacksonville, FL

Heart of gold: Actuarial opinion of a transplant
Stan Hines, MD, Huntsville, TX

Dukes of Hazard: Royal OSHA inspectors
Michael Kessler, MD, Houston, TX

Agony of defeat: Hammer toe
William M. Oppenhimer, MD, Houston, TX

Field of dreams: Psychoanalysis
Brett Johnson, MD, Erie, PA

Tons of fun: Jolly bariatric failure

> Bryon Labrenz, MD, Poughkeepsie, NY

Ball of wax: Otologist's dream

> Herbert Gersh, MD, Treasure Island, FL

Twist of fate: Spermatic cord torsion

> Douglas Ackerman, MD, Clackamas, OR

Point of no return: "Gimme those Metz," snapped the attending to the resident.

> Steve Lieberman, MD, Clackamas, OR

CITY CENTERS

ASSIGNMENT:
Alter the names of cities to make them medical meccas for specific specialized care.

EXAMPLES:
Buenos Aires (dentistry): Buenos Caries
Baton Rouge (alimentary): Baton Rugae
Khartoum (urology): Skrohtoum
Sevastopol (oncology): Seblastopol
Philadelphia (reimbursement): Billadelphia
Sacramento (psychiatry): Sacramental
Copenhagen (gynecology): Colpenhagen
Helsinki (fractures): Helslingi

ENTRIES:
Omsk (obstetrics): Momsk

Charles G. Eschenburg, MD, Delray Beach, FL

Kansas City (gastroenterology): Kansasacidity

Christopher W. Groner, MD, Jonesville, NC

Strasbourg (psychiatry): Stressbourg

Carl Sorgen, MD, Poughkeepsie, NY

Yonkers (psychiatry): Bonkers

Daniel J. Colombi, MD, Haddonfield, NJ

Casper (pulmonology): Gasper

Russell J. Cox, MD, Gastonia, NC

Bismarck (dermatology): Birthmarck

Gene Westveer, MD, Borculo, MI

Amityville (emergency medicine): Calamityville

Barni Schlein, Richmond, VA

El Paso (gastroenterology): El Gaso

Philip Paul, MD, Miami, FL

Juneau (gastroenterology): Jejuneau

Debi Robinson, San Diego, CA

London (pulmonology): Lungdom

Howard F. Neudorf, MD, Waipahu, HI

Jacksonville (orthopedics): Tractionville

Frank P. Reynolds, MD, Jacksonville, FL

Birmingham (parasitology): Wormingham

Floyd T. Nasuti, MD, Philadelphia, PA

Nashville (dermatology): Rashville

Steven Preston, MD, Harrisburg, PA

Caracas (forensic pathology): Carvacarcass

A. Sivakumar, MD, Henderson, NV

Haifa (mycology): Hyphae

Arthur N. Feinberg, MD, Kalamazoo, MI

Phoenix (doctors' reimbursement center): Feenix

Irving Thorne, MD, St. Louis Park, MN

Brest (cosmetic surgery): Greater Brest/Lesser Brest

J. Kennedy, DO, Fond du Lac, WI

Cairo (geriatrics): Medicairo

Kathy Waller, MD, Fort Collins, CO

Manila (gynecology): Monilia

Dr. Gary Blake, San Diego, CA

Stockholm (obstetrics): Storkhome

Douglas Ackerman, MD, Clackamas, OR

Nashville (oral surgery): Gnashville

Steven R. Drosman, MD, San Diego, CA

Lansing (surgery): Lancing

C. Alan Scott, MD, Marshall, MO

NOT QUITE TRITE

ASSIGNMENT:

Tailor a cliché so that its meaning has an application in the health care industry.

EXAMPLES:

A bolt from the blue—Spontaneous reversal of cyanosis
Down at the heels—The onset of plantar hirsutism
The whole ball of wax—View through the otoscope
Been around the block—Knows anesthesia
High five—The trigeminal nerve
Spare the rod—Preserve night vision
Ballpark figure—Habitus from overconsumption of peanuts and Cracker Jacks

ENTRIES:

Fit as a fiddle—Cello-shaped and seizing
Morey Filler, MD, San Francisco, CA

Stay the course—Don't skip out during CME classes.
James F. Gardner, MD, San Antonio, TX

Silence is golden—Cerumen impaction
Hugh H. Wang, MD, Concord, CA

At this point in time—A paper cut from news magazine
Robert C., Whitesitt, M.D., Helena, MT

Fly in the ointment—Emergency airlift of dermatology supplies
Steven Preston, MD, Harrisburg, PA

Cherchez la femme—All-male OB-GYN group in search of a patient
Daniel J. Colombi, MD, Haddonfield, NJ

It serves you right—A healed tennis elbow
Patrice J. Fogle, DO, Berea, KY

A blast from the past—Failed course of chemotherapy

William E. Somerall, Jr., MD, Birmingham, AL

Rotten apple—terrible case of laryngitis

Arumugam Sivakumar, MD, Henderson, NV

Take five—Transmetatarsal amputation

Melvin J. Breite, MD, Bayside, NY

A dime a dozen—New HMO fee schedule

Gerald E. Harris, MD, San Francisco, CA

When push comes to shove—Last few minutes of a delivery

Arthur S. Verdesca, MD, Morristown, NJ

Keep the change—Successful gender-altering operation

Ritchie C. Shoemaker, MD, Pokomoke City, PA

Much ado about nothing—Augmentation penoplasty.

S. D. Madduri, MD, Poplar Bluff, MO

Grin and bear it—Natural childbirth

Meyer B. Hodes, MD, East Rockaway, NY

Golden oldie—Jaundiced octogenarian

Gene Westveer, MD, Zeeland, MI

Nine cents short of a dime—Accepts capitation plans

Anthony J. Battista, MD, Stewart Manor, NY

A cut above the others—Successful surgeon

Edward M. Sessa, MD, Schenectady, NY

In the bag!—Successful orchiopexy

Ted McMahon, MD, Seattle, WA

True blue—Ultimate hypothermia

Stanley K. Rogers, DO, Oklahoma City, OK

What goes around comes around—Colonic fistula

Joseph B. Szgalsky, Woodbury, NJ

The long and short of it—Testbook chapter on pituitary disorders

Arthur N. Feinberg, MD, Kalamazoo, MI

Gutsy call—Phoning the patient's sigmoidoscopy results

Dan G. Severa, MD, Lawrence, KS

A trial balloon—The first angioplasty

Donald S. Brooks, MD, Redding, CA

The $64,000 question—Will Medicare cover the cost of my coronary bypass surgery?

Alan Solum, MD, Paynesville, MN

The whole nine yards—*Really* aggressive colonoscopy

Thomas J. Durkin, Jr., MD, Fort Washington, PA

Stan Hines, MD, Huntsville, TX

IN A WORD

ASSIGNMENT:

Convert a medical word phonetically into a complete nonmedical thought.

EXAMPLES:

"Urachus," rustled the amassed fallen leaves.

"Villi!" shouted the Swedish Nobelist-elect

"Cicatrix," grumbled the bored magic show viewer.

"Dystrophy . . . ," began the awarding league president.

ENTRIES:

"The cow he put in the barn and the occiput in the corral," said the Pennsylvania Dutchman.

Melvin J. Breite, MD, Bayside, NY

When I cauterize from across a crowded room, I knew it was love.

Steven Preston, MD, Harrisburg, PA

"Nomogram," mourned the elderly lady's bereaved family.

Alan L. Goldman, MD, Raleigh, NC

"Polymixin," whispered Long John Silver to his antisocial parrot.

Meyer B. Hodes, MD, East Rockaway, NY

Retina rage left Scarlett.

Gerry Lee Spooner, Mequon, WI

"Dysplasia far cry from the original novel," growled the cranky theater critic.

Anne Walker, MD, Charlotte, NC

"Rotator cuff," instructed her dressmaker to his assistant.

David M. Pease, MD, Estill, SC

"RU 486?" the confused mail carrier asked the householder.

Aileen Faulkner, Pittsburgh, PA

Pfannenstiehl is a heavy way to cool one's face.

Morey Filler, MD, San Francisco, CA

Finding a writing instrument, the traffic cop used appendicitis.

Robin Segal, Yardley, PA

Urinate sense of well-being is enviable.

Douglas Ackerman, MD, Clackamas, OR

"Anastomosis!" ordered a booming voice from heaven. "He needs one to ride to the Promised Land."

Robert L Hillary, MD, Findlay, OH

"Endophyte," pronounced the referee over the fallen boxer.

Daniel J. Colombi, MD, Haddonfield, NJ

"Floxin!" said the shepherd when the sheep came back.

John M. Cocco, MD, Valencia, CA

"Yaws," warned the Norwegian lifeguard.

Doris E. Fletcher, Kendall Park, NJ

"Dropsy from 'cup' and you get 'up,'" said the teacher.

Walter S. Mazen, Jr., MD, Chico, CA

"Barium enema study," commanded the Godfather.

Gene Westveer, MD, Zeeland, MI

"I'm innocent!" exclaimed the suspect. "You've got the rhonchi!"

Ted McMahon, MD, Seattle, WA

"Fundus!" demanded the researchers upon submission of their grant proposal.

Dave Taube, Oak Harbor, WA

Sandra Mamis, Poughkeepsie, NY

Paralyze: I didn't do it and I wasn't there.

Sue Pelinski, Park Ridge, IL

"Dysplastic," murmured the terrorist, selecting his explosives.

Peter J. Stahl, MD, Columbia, SC

Diverticulum: Scuba-related sexual harassment complaint.

Robert D. Lafsky, MD, Reston, VA

MERGERS

ASSIGNMENT:
Name the conglomerate that results when two or more medical entities come together.

EXAMPLES:
Dermatologist and investigative researcher: Hide-and-seek

Hypnotherapist and dentist: Trance and dental medication

Hematologist, dermatologist, and ophthalmologist: Blood, Sweat, and Tears

Neurologist, gastroenterologist, bowel surgeon, and gynecologist: Coma, colon, semicolon, period

Radiologist and rhinologist: The Shadow Nose

ENTRIES:
Acupuncturist and surgeon: Chinese takeout
> Kathy Waller, MD, Fort Collins, CO

Orthopedist and pediatrician: Bone à Petite
> Arthur E. LaMontagne, Jr., MD, Manchester, CT

Cardiac surgeon, hair transplanter, and pediatrician: CABG Patch Kids
> Daniel J. Colombi, MD, Haddonfield, NJ

Infectious diseases, dermatologist, obstetrician, and infertility: Rabies, Scabies, Tabes, Babies, and Maybes
> Michael Ichniowski, MD, Lutherville, MD

Otolaryngologist and orthopedist: Rhine-Os R Us
> Daniel Schual-Berke, MD, Seattle, WA

Bariatrician and psychiatrist: Mass hysteria
> Russell J. Cox, MD, Gastonia, NC

Radiologist, audiologist, and gynecologist: Film and sound reproductions
> Tejinder S. Sandhu, MD, Sanger, CA

Neurologist, infectious diseases, and audiologist: Tic, Tick, Tick-Tick

Morey Filler, MD, San Francisco, CA

Otolaryngologist and psychiatrist: *Scents and Sensibility*

Stephen Lieberman, MD, Clackamas, OR

Neurologist, orthopedist, and podiatrist: Tic, Tac, Toe

Robert L. Hillery, MD, Findlay, OH

Gerontologist, neonatologist, plastic surgeon, and pulmonologist: Something old, something new, something borrowed, something blue

James F. Gardner, MD, San Antonio, TX

Infertility specialist and ophthalmologist: The Egg and Eye

Alan L. Goldman, MD, Raleigh, NC

Ophthalmologist and urologist: *Field and Stream*

Doris E. Fletcher, Kendall Park, NJ

Irish and Jewish bowel surgeons: Kelly, Kelly, and Metzenbaum

Irving Thorne, MD, Bloomington, MN

Otologist, proctologist, psychiatrist, and utilization review organization: Ears, Rears, Fears, and Peers

Richard H. Bibler, MD, Pewaukee, WI

Dietitian and ophthalmologist: Weight and See

Steven Preston, MD, Harrisburg, PA

Orthopedist, pulmonologist, and chemical dependency specialist: Snap, Crackle, and Pop

Hugh Wang, MD, Concord, CA

Microbiologist, nuclear oncologist, pharmacist, and cardiologist: Prions and Geigers and Bayers, MI

Rachel Steinberg, Brooklyn, NY

CALL WAITING

ASSIGNMENT:
Convert a pager's signal to a sound or mode specific to the type of practitioner being summoned.

EXAMPLES:
Anesthesiologist—Zzzz
Allergist—Bee buzz
Physiatrist—No sound, just a vibrating massage

ENTRIES:
Family physician—Gate click

James T. Hay, MD, Del Mar, CA

Hernia surgeon—Bulge from beeper

Joseph B. Szgalsky, MD, Woodbury, NJ

Pediatrician—The beeper heats to 104 degrees

David A. Zomick, MD, Bristol, CT

Pulmonologist—Wind chimes

Ronald P. Olah, MD, Pasadena, CA

Obstetrician who is too late—Baby's cry

Allison Blomer, MD, Jensen Beach, FL

Pediatric orthopedist—Green stick snap and collie's bark

Dr. and Mrs. Thomas K. Rosvanis, Trafford, PA

Neurosurgeon—A slurping suction sound

Douglas Ackerman, MD, Clackamas, OR

Pathologist—First chords of Beethoven's Fifth Symphony

Stephen Lieberman, MD, Clackamas, OR

Urologist—Inflation of small perineal balloon

Arthur E. LaMontagne, Jr., MD, Manchesrter, CT

HMO doc—Any sound. Just wait seventy-two hours.

Stanley Rogers, DO, Oklahoma City, OK

ENT—Frog croak

Ralph French, MD, Anna Maria, FL

Psychiatrist—Primal scream

Paul J. Nuccio, MD, Tacoma, WA

Rheumatologist—Knuckles cracking

Laurel DeStefano, MD, Carmel, IN

Urologist—Short, cold squirt of quick-drying fluid

Tejinder S. Sandhu, MD, Sanger, CA

Pulmonologist—Smoke signals from beeper

Ronald P. Olah, MD, Pasadena, CA

Obstetrician, from patient in active labor—!#@!!*?##@@!!!**

Jerome M. Eder, MD, Agoura, CA

Electroencephalographer—Waves

Doris E. Fletcher, Kendall Park, NJ

Parasitolgist—*Tick-tick-tick*

Tejinder S. Sandhu, MD, Sanger, CA

Psychiatrist—Cuckoo, cuckoo

Multiple contributors

Reconstructive surgeon—*Ca-ching, ca-ching* (cash register)

Daniel J. Columbi, MD, Haddonfield, NJ

Neurologist—Tic Doc Tic Doc

Allan Plaut, MD, Lawrence, NY

HMO director—Same as immediately above

Melvin J. Breite, MD, Bayside, NY

Neurologist—Vibrations from a 256 tuning fork
Sandra Mamis, RPA-C, Poughkeepsie, NY

Internist—Hmmmm
Stan Hines, MD, Huntsville, TX

Urologist—Handel's Water Music Suite
Robert B. Quattlebaum, Jr., MD, Savannah, GA

Bariatrist—*Oink oink, oink oink*
Neal Green, MD, Corsicana, TX

GAFFES À LA WEBB

ASSIGNMENT:

Dr. C. W. Webb collects medical typos, misheard dictations, and malaprops, some of which are in the examples. Recall or compose a similar pratfall. Then add a comment or question that plays on it.

EXAMPLES:

Pulmonary vascular tour . . . unusual offering by travel agent?
Patient had no petal edema . . . and in the flower of his youth?
The femoral artery was closed shortly after his takeoff . . . bon voyage!
Patient had half a sister who had asthma . . . the other half is fine.

ENTRIES:

The patient complained of a spitting headache . . . keep your distance.

Irving Thorne, MD, Bloomington, MN

The artful breeder was controlled by cross-clamping . . . just where was that clamp?

William Zavod, MD, Merion, PA

He had a trick of Mona's infection . . . but his wife's name is Shirley!

Daniel J. Colombi, MD, Haddonfield, NJ

Patient got her ministration at sixteen . . . and was defrocked at seventeen.

Julio Novoa, MD, Lutherville, MD

I need a referral to that gastroentomologist . . . is it those butterflies again?

Meyer B. Hodes, MD, East Rockaway, NY

Examination of the neck revealed a brewery on the right . . . the left was cold sober.

Stan Hines, MD, Huntsville, TX

Hysteroscopy revealed mild endometrial hyperpleasure . . . a most enjoyable finding.

Steven Preston, MD, Harrisburg, PA

A myocardial infraction . . . for which he got a fifteen-yard penalty.

Frank P. Reynolds, MD, Jacksonville, FL

The patient has been under my car for two years . . . no wonder he's coughing.

Renee Katz, Bronx, NY

There was an erotic mummer present . . . a leftover from the Mardi Gras?

Ralph S. French, MD, Anna Maria, FL

Take one teaspoonful of metamutual . . . it's cheaper than Prudential.

Allan B. Solum, MD, Paynesville, MN

The patient has two brothers living and well; two sisters living in well . . . subterranean waterfront condo?

Cindi Ward, Rancho Mirage, CA

Trigamynal neuralgia . . . the pain of having three wives . . .

S. D. Madduri, MD, Poplar Bluff, MO

On lung exam, there were no crackles, rales, or weasels . . . hard to find, but always significant!

Meyer Ghen, MD, Bronx, NY

The patient had an incest bite . . . vacationing with his sister?

Diane Soares, Fall River, MA

We'll take the patient off diuretics and see how she dies . . . what if she does?

Gary J. Coomber, MD, Santa Rosa, CA

Hospital memo: The Infection Control Committee will meet on Thursday at noon to discuss sexually transmitted diseases on the floor . . . bed shortage?

Dan W. Chiles, MD, Placentia, CA

THE GOOD NEWS

ASSIGNMENT:
A punster delivers news of a high medical appointment. The beneficiary replies in kind.

EXAMPLES:
"The eyes have it. You've gotten the appointment." . . . ophthalmology . . . "Spec-macular!"

"The whealing and healing and dealing have paid off." . . . dermatology . . . "A sight for psoriasis!"

"All obstacles have been voided: Yerin!" . . . urology . . . "Urodynamic!"

ENTRIES:
"You lucky stiff, you're chief medical examiner." . . . pathology . . . "Be still, my beating heart!"

Steven Preston, MD, Harrisburg, PA

"Your new research appointment allows you to perform the rout of gout." . . . rheumatology . . . "Urica!"

Tejinder S. Sandhu, MD, Sanger, CA

"My encystence helped you worm your way into that one." . . . parasitology . . . "May they not put an ascaris by my name."

Russell J. Cox, MD, Gastonia, NC

"The board hopes that the delivery of this appointment is not premature." . . . obstetrics . . . "On the contrary, it's ultrasound!"

Alan L. Goldman, MD, Raleigh, NC

"The others bypassed the seat. Do you accept it?" . . . cardiology . . . "In a heartbeat!"

Walter S. Mazen, Jr., M.D., Chico, CA

"We need new blood to head the service. Will you do it?" . . . hematology . . . "Count me in."

A. E. Mgebroff, MD, Yoakum, TX

"Your predecessor was adept at stopping angioedema." . . . allergy . . . "He was a swell guy."

Leonard Schreier, MD, Bloomfield Hills, MI

"I got you the job because you're so articulate." . . . rheumatology . . . "It was a joint effort."

Linda LeMay, MD, Oneida, NY

"You've seized the title!" . . . neurology . . . "A fitting honor!"

C. M. McKenzie, Jr., MD, Columbia, SC

"Make no bones about it; we manipulated you into the job" . . . osteopathy . . . "Let's get cracking!"

Frank P. Reynolds, MD, Jacksonville, FL

"And so you have come to term with this crowning achievement." . . . obstetrics . . . "Inconceivable!"

James F. Gardner, MD, San Antonio, TX

"As chief, your first good break is to inaugurate the new lithotripter." . . . urology . . . "It's a real blast!"

Arthur E. LaMontagne, Jr., MD, Manchester, CT

"Congratulations, you've made the cut." . . . surgery . . . "Bloody good."

Herbert Gersh, MD, Treasure Island, FL

"You've accomplished such a feet by squeezing out a win for the chair." . . . podiatry . . . "It was really a shoe-in."

Brendan O. Duterte, MD, San Jose, CA

"The berth in our program is yours." . . . neonatology . . . "You must be kidding."

Leland Davis, MD, Santa Rosa, CA

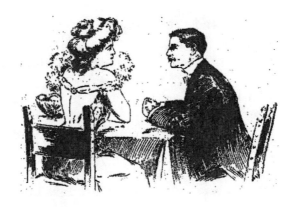

O CAPTION! MY CAPTION!

ASSIGNMENT:
Ascribe a suitable medical caption to the picture.

EXAMPLES:
"How long have you had this allergy to feathers?"
"I'm afraid you don't know what 'meeting your deductible' means."
"Your agent requires a bonus for signing with our clinic?"

ENTRIES:
"Don't despair, my dear Sigmund. It will get easier once Prozac is invented."

Margaret Bunger, MD, McLean, VA

"That's not quite what I meant when I asked you to put on a gown for your examinations."

Joseph B. Sgalsky, MD, Woodbury, NJ

"Okay, so I don't make more money than you do anymore. But I'm still the physician, I'm still your wife, and I'm still bigger than you!"

Hugh M. Wang, MD, Concord, CA

"Frankly, my dear, as your HMO director, I don't give a damn."

Arthur LaMontagne, Jr., MD, Manchester, CT
Similarly, Joel T Appleton, MD, Abilene, TX

"Oh yes, I often hold my consultations here: The duck a l'orange is superb and they have an allergy filter on their A/C."

Jackie Scoles, LPN and Lisa Line, LPN, Findlay, OH

"To answer your questions, sir, yes, I am indeed a fully trained urologist, and no, I cannot examine your prostate while you remain fully clothed and seated."

M. P. McCarthy, MD, Carlsbad, CA

"No, ma'am! I have no objection to female doctors at all . . . however, I seem to have forgotten what was ailing me."

Janie Niese, RN, Findlay, OH

"And another thing: for your hiatal hernia, wear only loose-fitting clothes."

Herbert Gersh, MD, Treasure Island, FL

"My dear, it's 1895—there are no rules yet regarding doctors dating patients."

Noelle M. Bothe, FNCP, Houston, TX

"Please, Victoria, you always get to play the nurse. When do I get my turn?"

Daniel Schual-Berke, MD, Seattle, WA

"I am afraid this dinner is not a covered benefit."

Irving Thorne, MD, St. Louis Park, MN

"Confidentially, Phen-Fen helped me get into this old dress."

Roger H. Wang, MD, Santa Ana, CA

Similarly, J. Marc Rosen, MD, Waianae, HI

"I would love to get up and dance with you, dear, but you're stepping on my catheter line."

Lawrence K. Harris, MD, Reading, PA

IN DISMISSAL MODE

ASSIGNMENT:
How best can a medical colleague be told to leave? By specialty, of course. Use directness.

EXAMPLES:
Bacteriologist—"Bug off."
Nuclear internist—"Fall out."
Surgeon—"Cut out!"
Dermatologist—"Flake off."

ENTRIES:
Hematologist—"Outocyte!"

Arthur N. Feinberg, MD, Kalamazoo, MI

Hearing specialist—"Audios, amigo!"

David P. Perkins, MD, Huntingdon Valley, PA

Oncologist—"BCNU."

Vincent L. Keipper, MD, Concord, NC

TB specialist—"Get ghon."

Glenn H. Perelson, MD, Bonita, CA

Podiatrist—"Shoe!"

Chitra Radhakrishnan, Dix Hills, NY

Psychiatrist—"DSMiss yourself!"

Hyman J. Milstein, MD, Studio City, CA

Hepatologist—"Bye-all."

Allan Plant, Lawrence, NY

Orthopedist—"Hasta lumbago."

Steven Lieberman, MD, Clackamas, OR

Cloning specialist—"Depart on the double."

Kathy Waller, MD, Fort Collins, CO

Industrial medicine specialist—"Punch out!"

David Brody, DMD, Lafayette, NJ

House staff resident—"You're history."

Ralph S. French, MD, Anna Maria, FL

Gastroenterologist—"May the wind always be at your back."

Daniel J. Colombi, MD, Haddonfield, NJ

Cardiologist—"You're ejected."

W. E. Watkins, M.D., Nampa, ID

Medical ethicist—"Why don't you take the high road?

Thomas J. Durkin, Jr., MD, Fort Washington, PA

Ophthalmologist—"sEe you."

Edward M. Sessa, MD, Schenectady, NY

Chest surgeon—"Get crackin'!"

Bernard Greenberg, MD, Tucker, GA

Trauma surgeon—"Hit the road."

David A. Miller, MD, Wildwood, MO

Gastroenterologist—"Evacuate."

Daniel Sporn, Athens, PA

Pulmonologist—"Blow!"

H. Bennett, MD, Washington, DC

Dermatologist—"Break out!"

Janice Ducksworth, Chicago, IL

Obstetrician—"Head out."

Debra Walland, MD, Wakefield, RI

Hypnotist—"Remove yourself from here."

Joel D. Lilly, MD, Seattle, WA

Rheumatologist—"Blow the joint.'

Stephen L. Kaufman, MD, San Francisco, CA

Pediatrician—"Toddle away."

Russell J. Cox, MD, Gastonia, NC

Cryotherapist—"Chill out."

Howard F. Neudorf, MD, Waipahu, HI

Obstetrician—"Abort."

Grafton C. Fanney, Jr., MD, Euclid, OH

Sleep therapist—"Good night."

Allan B. Solum, MD, Paynesville, MN

Laser surgeon—"Evaporate."

William Zavod, MD, Merion, PA

A STEP BEYOND

ASSIGNMENT:
Since bigness is in vogue, enlarge medical words in megalomaniac fashion.

EXAMPLES:
Truckbunkle—An industrial-sized abscess
Megalithotripsy—All day in the tub
Papal ligament—The ultimate uterine support
Grandpopliteal—The father of all fossae
Grandmalpractice—A case that befits lawyers prone to maximal seizure

ENTRIES:
Cardinal Cushing—Suprasuprarenal function
Irving Thorne, MD, St. Louis Park, MN

Astrodomocytoma—An outsized brain tumor
Tejinder S. Sandhu, MD, Sanger, CA

Polyanaphylaxis—Exaggerated allergic response in irrepressibly optimistic subjects
Joseph F. J. Curi, MD, Torrington, CT

Eightceps—Perfect for the delivery of twins
Morey Filler, MD, San Francisco, CA

Cardinal synapse—Transgressor transmitter
G. E. Ristow, DO, East Lansing, MI

BeTen—Absolute certainty of nonmalignant state
Mark Saylor, MD, Topeka, KS

Big macular—Rash following excessive fast-food ingestion
Floyd T. Nasuti, MD, Philadelphia, PA

Dinopsoriasis—Skin affliction with huge scales.
Alan Goldman, MD, Raleigh, NC

Knee plus ultra—Tops in sprains
Ralph S. French, MD, Anna Maria, FL

TIGER scan—Imagery for gigantic patients
Alan B. Solum, MD, Paynesville, MN

Triabetes—Now with three times the sugar!
Steven Preston, MD, Harrisburg, PA

Colossustrum—Baby's first supersized drink
Gary J. Colombert, MD, Santa Rosa, CA

Supercalifragilisticosteoporosis—Extra-brittle bones.
M. B. Price, MRN, Gonzalez, TX

Watermelonoma—Tumor removable by Mohs megagraphic technique
Gene Westveeer, MD, Zeeland, MI

Magnumbness—Hypoesthesia with excessive tippling
Stan Hines, MD, Huntsville, TX

Gallonan fever—Most diaphoretic form of malaria
Kathy Waller, MD, Flort Collins, CO

Anal gorge—A really big fissure
Ronald P. Olah, MD, Pasadena, CA

Latexas allergy—*Large* reaction to latex
Joseph B. Szgalsky, MD, Woodbury, NJ

Humongustatory belch—Long, loud, without class
Hugh H. Wang, MD, Concord, CA

Rolypolyhydramnios—So much amniotic fluid you can't walk
Neal Green, MD, Corsicana, TX

The big leioma—More than just a fib roid
Daniel J. Colombi, MD, Haddonfield, NJ

Gargantuenteritis—A *big* tummyache

Herbert Gersh, MD, Treasure Island, FL

King Colonoscope—indicated for megacolons

Karen K. Nellis, R.N., Frederick, MD

Ins-pectoralis major—Head of the Division of Plastic Surgery.

Arthur E. LaMontagne, Jr., MD, Manchester, CT

Quinti-, septi-, octiceps—muscular results of steroid overdosage

Julio Novoa, MD, Lunterville, MD

AT THE BRINK

ASSIGNMENT:
With what last words would those of the medical fraternity step into the Great Beyond?

EXAMPLES:
Podiatrist: "On my immortal sole . . ."
Immunologist: "That oncoming car! I hope I'm autoimmune . . ."
Orthopedist: "I repair to a higher joint . . ."
Obstetrician: "Your baby is really ugly . . ."
Psychiatrist: "Paranoid, yes, but I never took you to be homici—"

ENTRIES:
Hand surgeon: "I think I'm losing my grip."

Stan Hines, MD, Huntsville, TX

Urologist: "Alas, I'm going from prostate to prostrate."

Russell M. Sacco, MD, Lake Oswego, OR

Microbiologist: "Look, don't you think I can tell the difference between Ebola and E. coli?"

Steven Preston, MD, Harrisburg, PA

Urologist: I guess I'll go with the flow."

Lenore C. Deeths, Omaha, NE

Proctologist: (*Gasp*) "I never realized the end was so near!"

Daniel Schual-Berke, M.D., Seattle, WA

Oncologist: "A.P.O.P.T.O . . . S . . . I . . . S . . ."

Jerome M. Eder, MD, Agoura, CA

HMO CEO: Of course, He'll approve me for a longer stay on earth."

Alan L. Goldman, MD, Raleigh, NC

Radiation oncologist: "Beam me up."

James F. Gardner, MD, San Antonio, TX

Medical school professor: "One last pearl before the gates close . . ."

Charles G. Eschenburg, MD, Delray Beach, FL

Sex therapist: "Me Tarzan, you Jane."

Melvin J. Breite, MD, Bayside, NY

HMO administrator: "It is a far, far better thing I do . . ."

Joel T. Appleton, MD, Abilene, TX

Urologist: "No, I'm not giving you the finger."

Barbara Starr, Encino, CA

Any MD: "I worked in an HMO, so hell should be an upgrade."

Daniel J. Colombi, MD, Haddonfield, NJ

Oral surgeon: "Vlad, unusually large cuspids . . ."

Robert W. Sellers, MD, Fleetwood, PA

Sports medicine specialist: "I hope this event is the high jump."

Sue Kornack, RN, Findlay, OH

Pediatrician: "Yes, your baby doesn't look right, but did you ever see yourself in the mirror?"

Floyd T. Nasuti, MD, Philadelphia, PA

Plastic surgeon: "Please, take my business card. If anyone ever needed it, you sure—"

April Ritter-Hoffman, LPN, Charleston, WV

Urologist: "I have to go."

Donald Barkan, MD, Swampscott, MA

Microbiologist: "You mean it was not mustard, just a botulism culture?"

A. Zambra, MD, Houston, TX

Cardiologist: "Be still my heart."

Michael J. Zappitelli, D.O., Norristown, PA

Otolaryngologist: "Say AAAAARGH!"

Dan Steinbrocker, Los Angeles, CA

IN THE BEGINNING

ASSIGNMENT:
Provide a name for the opening rites of a medical, or medically related, facility.

EXAMPLES:
Neonatal hospital—Preemiere
Ophthalmology—Eye-opener
Psychiatry—Head start
General surgery—Grand opening
Hematology—First blood
Radiology—Pre-view

ENTRIES
Surgery—A black tie event

Chuck J. Cucchiara, MD, Matairie, LA

Obstetrics—Induction and cord-cutting

Paul T. Gunderson, MD, Manistee, MI

Brain surgery—Galea opening

Gene Westveer, MD, Zeeland, MI

Psychiatry—Primal scream

Arthur N. Feinberg, MD, Kalamazoo, MI

Endocrinology—Gland opening

Douglas Ackerman, MD, Clackamas, OR

Lithotripsy—Big bang

Tejinder S. Sandhu, MD, Sanger, CA

Ophthalmology—Grand myopening

S. D. Madduri, MD, Poplar Bluff, MO

Hematology-oncology—Blastoff

Irving Thorne, MD, St. Louis Park, MN

Urology—Seminal session

Neal M. Fallis, MD, Westborough, MA

Obstetrics—First presentation

Thomas Lee Bucky, MD, Weston, CT

Brachytherapy—Preseeding operations

Brian S. Moran, MD, Hinsdale, IL

Taxpayer-sponsored laser surgicenter—Toasting the citizens

William G. White, MD, Franklin Park, IL

Dermatology—Skinitiation

Steven Preston, MD, Harrisburg, PA

Microbiology lab—Cellabration

Thomas R. White, MD, St. Petersburg, FL

Obstetrics—Heeere it comes!

Julio C. Novoa, MD, Baltimore, MD

Nuclear medicine—Up and atom

David Perkins, MD, Huntington Valley, PA

Cryogenics lab—Ice breaker

Michael Leonard, MD, Binghamton, NY

Gynecology—Maiden voyage

Bernard Greenberg, MD, Decatur, GA

Gynecology—Initial pubic offering

James F. Gardner, MD, San Antonio, TX
Similarly, Arthur E. LaMontagne, MD,
Manchester, CT

Sleep disorder clinic—First night

Joseph F. J. Curi, MD, Torrington, CT

Obesity clinic—The start of something big
Kathy Waller, MD, Fort Collins, CO

Pediatrics—New kid on the block
Howard Neudorf, MD, Waipahu, HI

Neurologist, neurosurgeon—Opening sellabration
Doris Fletcher, Kendall Park, NJ Morey Filler, MD, San Francisco, CA

MOTTOROLA (suggested by Gene C. Lawrence, MD)

ASSIGNMENT:
Create a motto for a practice, suitable for letterheads, business cards, or media spots.

EXAMPLES:
Cardiology: "Facing our tracing is bracing."
Plastic Surgery: "Where all graft is on the level."
Urology: "Write yourself a bill of health at our Watermen's pen."
Obstetrics: "No fetus can beat us."

ENTRIES:
Infectious diseases: "Medical care with culture and sensitivity."

Hal B. Jenson, MD, San Antonio, TX

Geriatrics: "We provide care for the elderly, don't we?"

Richard A. Mahrer, MD, San Jose, CA

Canadian infectious disease specialist: "O Candida."

Douglas Ackerman, MD, Clackamas, OR

Thyroid clinic: "You can come to our port in a storm."

Alan L. Goldman, MD, Raleigh, NC

Neurosurgery: "We treat your cranium like uranium."

Linda Lemay, MD, and Scott Treatman, MD,
Cazenovia, NY

Plastic Surgery: "If it ain't broke, we fix it."

Renee Salvino, MD, Prospect Heights, IL

Lithotripsy: "Have gun, makes gravel."

James F. Gardner, MD, San Antonio, TX

Laser surgery: "We love to fry and it shows."

> Arthur E. LaMontagne, Jr., MD, Manchester, CT
> Steven Preston, MD, Harrisburg, PA

Psychiatry: "We love to pry and it shows."

> Steven Preston, MD, Harrisburg, PA

Pulmonary medicine: "Every little wheeze seems to whisper disease."

> Jeffrey K. Pearson, DO, San Marcos, CA

Lithotripsy: "You'll love our heated indoor pool."

> Kathy Waller, MD, Fort Collins, CO

Malpractice attorney: "Veni, vidi, victim."

> Paul J. Nuccio, MD, Tacoma, WA

Obstetrics: "We're the light at the end of the tunnel."

> Beverly Sykes, Davis, CA

Internal medicine: "Precise diagnosis despite your neurosis."

> William M. Simons, MD, Lake Worth, FL

Urology (impotence): "We start with a three-to-four inch floppy . . ."

> Morey Filler, MD, San Francisco, CA

Urology (impotence): "Nowadays a hard man is good to find."

> William V. Adler, MD, Downey, CA

Oncology: "We're chemo-savvy."

> Anthony Somkin, MD, Berkeley, CA

Hepatology: "We de liver."

> Melvin J. Breite, MD, Bayside, NY

Dietitian: "If you're thick and tired . . ."

> Jay Malhotra, MD, Homewood, IL

Geriatric urologist: "Gently down your stream."

> Barnaby F. Starr, MD, Baltimore, MD

BABY TALK

ASSIGNMENT:
Pick a name for a baby whose parents have specific aspirations in health care for the newborn.

EXAMPLES:
Flossie—dental technician
Imogene—X-ray technician
Maximillian—HMO CEO
Bertha—Obstetrician

ENTRIES:
Sinbad—Venereologist

Kathy Waller, MD, Ft. Collins, CO

Millicent—HMO executive in charge of physician reimbursement

Russell Cox, MD, Gastonia, NC

Ramsey—Colonoscopist

Daniel J. Colombi, MD, Haddonfield, NJ

Cokie—Substance abuse expert

Allan R. LaReau, MD, Kalamazoo, MI

Manuel—Hand surgeon

Tejinder S. Sandhu, MD, Sanger, CA

Jules—Urologist

Steven Lieberman, MD, Clackamas, OR

Electra—EKG technician

A. Zambra, MD, Houston, TX

Boris—Statistician

Charles G. Eschenburg, MD, Delray Beach, FL

Buddy—Mycologist

Philip Paul, MD, Miami, FL

Barb—Phlebotomist

Arthur E. LaMontagne, Jr., MD, Manchester, CT

Bridget—Dental prosthetist

Doris E. Fletcher, Kendall Park, NJ

Fillmore—Dentist

Douglas Ackerman, MD, Clackamas, OR

Les—HMO precertifier

Jonathan Ehrlich, MD, Atlanta, GA

Horst—Laryngologist

William G. White, MD, Franklin Park, IL

Melanie—Dermatologist

Dr. William Zavod, Merion, PA

Borg—Gastroenterologist

Gary M. Gorlick, MD, Los Angeles, CA

Van—Ambulance driver

Suzanne Hollander, MD, San Diego, CA

Rex—Pharmacist

Aviva Nazbatian, RN, Manhasset Hills, NY

Adeline—Chiropractor

S. J. Hirsh, MD, Chester, PA

Flora—Infectious disease specialist

Kiran A. Majmundar, MD, Charleston, WV

Drew—Phlebotomist

Robert L. Hillery, MD, Findlay OH

Caesar—Obstetrician

Multiple contestants

Pearl—Internist at teaching hospital

Jacob Skezas, MD, Ithaca, NY

Mort—Pathologist

Arthur N. Feinberg, MD, Kalamazoo, MI

Candida—Microbiologist

Lynette J. Mazur, MD, Houston, TX

Twins Sylvia and Rolando—Neurologists

Alton R. Prihoda, MD, Baytown, TX

Felix Sigmund—Endoscopist

Gene Westveer, MD, Zeeland, MI

Chester—Pulmonologist

Richard D. Shafron, MD, Hollywood, FL

HANG YOUR HAT

ASSIGNMENT:
Create an appropriately named venue at which a health care professional plies his/her trade.

EXAMPLES:
Allergist—Wheezy Street
Medical examiner—Boardway
Gastroenterologist—Avenue of the Entericas

ENTRIES:
Psychiatrist—Pick-a-Dilly Square
Joseph B. Szgalsky, MD, Woodbury, NJ

Alternative medicine—Second Avenue
Joseph Grayzel, MD, Englewood, NJ

Gynecologist—St. D
Dave Taube, Oak Harbor, WA

Endodontist—Root 66
James Tate, MD, Kokomo, IN

Gastroenterologist—Magenstrasse
Rudi Kirschner, MD, Phoenix, AZ

Oriental nutritionist—Vi-Ta-Minh Trail
Joseph F. J. Curi, MD, Torrington, CT

HMO executive—Rue de la Pay
Daniel J. Colombi, MD, Haddonfield, NJ

Biochemist—Beaker Street
Doris E. Fletcher, Kendall Park, NJ

Neonatology—Dearborn Avenue
E. U. and E. M. Herrero, MD, Southgate, MI

Psychiatrist—Boulevard of Spoken Dreams

Benjamin Kendall, MD, Wynnewood, PA

Any endoscopist—The Throughway

Tom Savoie, D.O., Huntington, IN

Breast surgeon—Mammorial Drive

Jay Malhotra, MD, Homewood, IL

Cardiologist—Starling Curve

David Perkins, MD, Huntington Valley, PA

Pediatrician—Malibubu Highway

Russell Cox, MD, Gastonia, NC

Brain surgeon—Neural Block

Pamela Markovich, EMT, Scarsdale, NY

Infectious disease specialist—Tetracyc Lane

Douglas Ackerman, MD, Clackamas, OR

Dentist—Chomps-Elysées

Julie Schilling, Easton, MD

Urology—The Exstressway

Richard N. Levrault, DO, Canton, MA

Orthopedist—Sesamoid Street

Magdelyn Sabichi, MD, Denver, CO

Dermatologist—B'wartway at Pock Place

Allan Plaut, MD, Lawrence, NY

Dermatologist—Hide Park

Vicente E. Velasco, MD, Glendale, AZ

Obstetrician—Chorionic Villa

George G. Imrie, MD, Thornton, NH

Mammoplasty specialist—Frontage Road

Ted McMahon, MD, Seattle, WA

Cardiologist—The Pauseway

R. Schlein, MD, Richmond, VA

Sex therapist—Forty-seconds Street

Steven Preston, MD, Harrisburg, PA

Radiation oncologist—Rad Square

Arthur E. LaMontagne, Jr., MD, Mancnester, CT

SPELL CHECK

ASSIGNMENT:
Remove a letter from a medical word, substitute one or more letters, producing a new word with an imaginative definition

EXAMPLES:
Flic douloureaux—A sad movie
Stoxsackie—Investment portfolio
Sternup—A dire maritime state
Godad—Exhortation at senior's track meet

ENTRIES
Hematocrisp—Iron-rich cereal

David A. Kline, MD, Los Angeles, CA

Chicken lox—Smoked salmon afraid of swimming upstream

Morey Filler, MD, San Francisco, CA

Trigaminal neuralgia—Pain of having three wives

Sivaprasad D. Madduri, Poplar Bluff, MO

Puckwickian syndrome—Disease of obese hockey players

Joseph B. Szgalsky, MD, Woodbury, NJ

Slammer toe—Malady of inmates' feet

Ronald Olah, MD, Pasadena, CA

Gaulimia—Insatiable indulgence in French cuisine

Joseph F. J. Curi, MD, Torrington, CT

Beswign—What piglets aspire to

Douglas Ackerman, MD, Clackamas, OR

Facteria—Manufacturing site for bacteriological weapons

Tejinder S. Sandhu, MD, Sanger, CA

Fetastasis—Spoiled cheese

J. D. Smith, MD, West Hartford, CT

Teniscus—Exclamation after missing an easy overhead

Alan Goldman, MD, Raleigh, NC

Otoslope—A decline in hearing

Stephen Lieberman, MD, Clackamas, OR

Lupus bulgaris—Wolf from the Balkans

Steven S. Spencer, MD, Sevierville, TN

Bunter's canal—Between pitcher and third base

Daniel J. Colombi, MD, Haddonfield, NJ

Organic grain syndrome—Illness from natural causes

Richard A. Mahrer, MD, San Jose, CA

Pop smear—Familiar stain on children's clothing

Robert Resnick, MD, Fokrest Hills, NY

Wormulary—A collection of usage standards for bait shops

Tom Savoie, DO, Huntington, IN

Morbelliform—Consequence of dietary excess

William T. Zempsky, MD, West Hartford, CT

Triphlegminal—When polite throat-clearing doesn't get attention

Jay Malhotra, MD, Homewood, IL

Barborygmi—Rumblings in the tavern

Doris E. Fletcher, Kendall Park, NJ

Irritable vowel syndrome—"Say 'aah', dammit!"

Scott Treatman, DO, and Linda Lemay, MD,
Cazenovia, NY

Jestation—Pregnancy with a future comedian

R. Schlein, MD, Richmond, VA

Goobernaculum—A nutty means of support

> Stanley J. K. Rogers, DO, Oklahoma City, OK

Erection fraction—Rating scale for older men

> Bernadine Z. Paulshock, MD, Wilmington, DE

Varicello—A blistering string solo

> F. Malkin, MD, Whittier, CA

Corpus delicio—Cannibal cordon bleu dinner

> Morris Spielberg, MD, Brooklyn, NY

Servix—Restaurant employee (female form of "server")

> Charles W. Webb, MD, Traverse City, MI

Berruca—A Hebrew prayer about a wart

> Glenn S. Sherman, MD, Macungie, PA

Castric ulcer—Stress ulcer stemming from fear of being castrated

> Daniel Schual-Berke, MD, Seattle, WA

IN CONCERT

ASSIGNMENT:
Select a classical musical opus and ascribe to it a medical spin-off.

EXAMPLES:
Academic Festival—Yearly meeting of the American College
The Nutcracker—Craniotomy
Pathetique—Caregivers' inevitably futile plea to DSHS for reimbursement
Carnival of the Animals—Malpractice lawyers' convention

ENTRIES:
Candide—Honest admission of one's yeast infection
Vicente E. Velasco III, MD, Glendale, AZ

The Four Seasons—Medicare, HMOs, PPOs, empty office
Jay Malhotra, MD, Homewood, IL

Eine Kleine Nachtmusik—Need for an adenoidectomy
Rudy Kirschner, MD, Phoenix, AZ

Rondo in B-sharp—Ward rounds with the chief of service
Melvin J. Breite, MD, Bayside, NY

Dance of the Comedians—Peer review committee
Leonard W. Rozin, MD, Oklahoma City, OK

Falstaff—Needing a urologist
Edward Lamon, MD, Albuquerque, NM

Peter and the Wolf—Dual certification in urology and eating disorders
Anne E. Walker, MD, Matthews, NC

Dance of the Hours—A phone call to Blue Cross
David A. Kline, MD, Los Angeles, CA

"The Minute Waltz"—What's left of patient care after fulfilling Medicare's coding and documentation requirements

Joseph B. Szgalsky, MD, Woodbury, NJ

The Emperor's Clothes—Tailored scrub suits for the chief of surgery

Joseph F. J. Curi, MD, Torrington, CT

Ode to Joy—Vindication in a malpractice case

Howard S. Goldberg, MD, Southfield, MI

Julio C. Novoa, MD, Perry Hall, MD

La Sonnambula—Obstetrician whose only associate is on holiday

Daniel J. Colombi, MD, Haddonfield, NJ

The Golden Peacock—HMO top CEO

A. Zambra, MD, Houston, TX

Rage Over a Lost Penny—Response to another cut in the fee schedule

David A. Herzog, MD, New Rochelle, NY

Boris Godunov—A soporific anatomy professor

Eleanor Calhoun, Staten Island, NY

The Magic Flute—A penile prosthesis

James Kline, MD, St. Joseph, MO

Three Pieces—A good result, according to Humpty Dumpty's HMO

Stan Hines, MD, Huntsville, TX

The Thieving Magpie—Fraudulent Medicare provider

Robert B. Bux, MD, London, KY

L'Elisir D'Amore—Viagra

Morris Spielberg, MD, Brooklyn, NY

Kaisermarsch—Mass exodus of primary care doctors from large HMO

Teresa Brock, MD, Clayton, CA

SANGFROID

ASSIGNMENT:

Cause the patient, en route to the operating room, to toss off an anxiety-relieving bon mot.

EXAMPLES:

D & C: "I've been through worse scrapes than this."
Craniotomy: "This hasn't been a good hair day."
Knee arthroscopy: "This could be ex-cruciating."
Varicose veins: "I can't wait to see the stripper."
Femoral neck repair: "This is a hip-pinning happening."

ENTRIES:

Extraction delivery: "May the forceps be with you, Obie."
Jonathan H. Rosen, MD, Bristol, CT

Mammary implants: "I'm hoping all goes well. I'm hoping all goes well."
Bernadine Z. Paulshock, MD, Wilmington, DE

Cesarean section: "But I'm not Italian!"
Joel T. Appleton, MD, Abilene, TX

Circumcision: "Let's cut to the chase and not talk about my shortcomings."
Ingrid and James Beckett, MD, Davis, CA

Circumcision: "This downsizing has gone too far."
Morris Spielberg, MD, Brooklyn, NY

Circumcision: "Spare the rod."
James Tate, MD, Kokomo, IN

Penile prosthesis: "I guess I'm getting my comeuppance."
A. P. Rockwood, MD, Fredericksburg, TX

Splenectomy: "I need to vent."

R. Schlein, MD, Richmond, VA

Siamese twins separation: "See y'all later, I gotta split."

Robert R. Jones, MD, Nevada, MO

Pacemaker implantation: "Your pace or mine?"

Steven G. Hull, MD, Overland Park, KS

Hernia repair: "I guess duct tape won't do."

Arman H. Arslanian, MD, Rome, GA

Laser dermatology: "Cleared for takeoff."

Barbara Starr, MFCC, Encine, CA

Recurrent hernia repair: "Don't mesh with me."

Jay Malhotra, MD, Homewood, IL

Craniotomy: "Is this procedure covered under capitation?"

April Ritter-Hoffman, LPN, Charleston, WV

Hemorrhoidectomy: "The end justifies the means."

Robert C. Whitesitt, MD, Helena, MT

Renal stone removal: "How good are you at calculus?"

Russell J. Cox, MD, Gastonia, NC

Vovulus repair: "I guess I won't be kinky anymore."

William A. Sinton, MD, Towson, MD

Phalloplasty: "I'm going to go straight after this."

Edward Joseph, MD, Monticello, KY

Prostatectomy: "I'd rather pee in Philadelphia."

Meyer Hodes, MD, Oceanside, NY

Pneumonectomy: "Out, out damned spot."

Morey Filler, MD, San Francisco, CA

TITULAR

ASSIGNMENT:
Choose an unofficial title or nickname after some celebrity and ascribe it to an individual of some health care pursuit. Said title or nickname can be slightly altered. Celebrity need not be real.

EXAMPLES:
Plastic surgeon—Der Alterer (Konrad Adenauer)
Sports physician—The Sultan of Sweat (Babe Ruth)
Department head—The Lady in the Chair (Cassiopeia)
Rough surgeon—Old Blood and Guts (General George Patton)

ENTRIES:
Chief of invasive cardiology—First in the hearts of his countrymen (George Washington)

Bernadine Z. Paulshock, MD, Wilmington, DE

Mayo Clinic dietitian—Minnesota Fats (Rudolf Wanderone)

Daniel J. Colombi, MD, Haddonfield, NJ

Soviet contrast manufacturer—The Red Barium (Baron Manfred von Richtofen)

Stan Hines, MD, Huntsville, TX

Petit mal specialist—Little Seizure (Edward G. Robinson)

William V. Adler, MD, Downey, CA

Family practitioner in an HMO—the Gate-ist (Muhammad Ali)

Bill Garvin, DO, Easton, MD

Sex change surgeon—The Maleman (Karl Malone)

Douglas Ackerman, MD, Clackamas, OR

New England circumciser—The Yankee Clipper (Joe DiMaggio)

Herbert Gersh, MD, Treasure Island, FL
Similarly, Douglas R. Eisenstein, DO, Tucson, AZ

Electroshock therapist—Joltin' Joe (Joe DiMaggio)

Vincent L. Keipper, MD, Concord, NC

Vascular surgeon—Man of Steal (Clark Kent/Superman)

Jay Malhotra, MD, Homewood, IL

ENT group—The Four Hoarsemen (Notre Dame's Miller, Layden, Crowley, and Stuhldreher)

Roland P. Olah, MD, Pasadena, CA

Allergist—A Man for All Seasons (Sir Thomas More)

R. Schlein, MD, Richmond, VA

Epidemiologist—The Hunter (Orion)

Russell J. Cox, MD, Gastonia, NC

Forceps-wielding obstetrician—Sitting Pull (Sioux chief)

Julio C. Novoa, MD, Perry Hall, MD

Dermatologist—King of Pop (Michael Jackson)

John C. Knight, MD, Huntsville, TX

GRAVE UNDERTAKING

ASSIGNMENT:
Create an epitaph in couplet form that identifies the deceased's medical pursuit.

EXAMPLES:
Neurologist: He cased the cord and foiled the fit
At least till his synapses quit.

Urologist: TURPs done, he's now been sadly cast
Beneath a stone he cannot blast.

Internist: He was a whiz at diagnosis
Until he underwent necrosis.

Pathologist: He diagnosed from slides a-million
Till transferred to his own pavilion.

ENTRIES:
Laryngologist: He healed aphonia; at cords he poked
One winter's day, 'twas he who croaked.

Meyer B. Hodes, MD, East Rockaway, NY

Allergist: After years of shots, it's only just
That now he's turned to mold and dust.

Alan L. Goldman, MD, Raleigh, NC

Medical malpractice expert: He would have been a saint if
He hadn't argued for the plaintiff.

Daniel J. Colombi, MD, Haddonfield, NJ

Gynecologist: She was a whiz with things follicular
Whizless since unperpendicular.

Stanley Rogers, DO, Oklahoma City, OK

Insurance company CEO: "My HMO rules I deserve," he cried,
"Immortal life." Claim denied.

Jonathan Ehrlich, MD, Atlanta, GA

Transplant surgeon: Heart, liver, kidney, to others he granted.
Now here he lies—he's been transplanted

Carolyn Smith, Mercer Island, WA

Oncologist: From malign immortal diagnosis
His cells are all in apoptosis.

W. D. Bailey, MD, College Station, TX

Radiologist: He read a lot of X-ray pics
Until he crossed the river Styx.

Patrick M. Boccagno, MD, Altoona, PA

Plastic surgeon: Strengthened jawlines, straightened noses . . .
All for naught, he's feeding roses.

Joel Schwartzberg, Maplewood, NJ

Oncologist: She warned her patients not to smoke
Yet smoking made the warner croak.

Joseph Szgalsky, MD, Woodbury, NJ

Orthopedist: He mended others' bones with bliss
But never braced himself for this!

Tom Savoie, DO, Huntington, IN

Managed-care primary physician: He served his time as the gatekeeper
But could not hide from the Grim Reaper.

G. J. Billmeier, Jr., MD, Memphis, TN

Psychiatrist: Relations healed and psyches mended
The moods are up, but his own wit's ended.

Gene Westveer, MD, Zeeland, MI

Endocrinologist: Thyroid nodules he did needle
Extra time he could not wheedle.

Philip Schmidt, MD, Brooklyn, NY

Aerospace MD: In life his feats all folks astounded
Alas, he is forever grounded.

Robert L. Hillery, MD, Findlay, OH

Plastic surgeon: Ashes to ashes, dust to dust
I've augmented my final bust.

David Taube, Oak Harbor, WA

Pulmonologist: She treated ev'ry wheeze and rale
Till sadly she ceased to inhale.

Diana Lowenthal, MD, Valhalla, NY

Urologist: He lies 'neath stone, the Cysto Kid
He helped 'em void is what he did.

W. E. Watkins, MD, Nampa, ID

SPORTING MOVES

ASSIGNMENT:
Medically redefine a procedure or maneuver in a well-known sport.

EXAMPLES:
Pick and roll: Method of patient transfer from OR table
Overhead smash: Cause of subdural hematoma
Squeeze play: Decision to avoid Cesarean Section
Single wing formation: Preparation of unilateral splint and sling
Hitting short of the green: Being denied payment by insurer

ENTRIES:
Slam dunk: Hydrotherapy for the noncompliant
Ron Pennington, MD, Newport Beach, CA

Baltimore chop: Amputation at Johns Hopkins
Joseph F. J. Curi, MD, Torrington, CT

Roughing the passer: Painful kidney stone
Ron Sklar, MD, Portland, OR

Grand slam: What happens to a resident after presenting a disaster at M&M
Douglas Ackerman, MD, Clackamas, OR

Four-bagger: Aggressive treatment for dehydration
Allan R. LaReau, MD Vicksburg, MI

Lap the field: Explore the abdomen
Robert Edelman, MD, Garden City, NY

Interference: Your request for authorization has been denied by HMO.
Jeffrey J. Rabinovitz, MD, Placerville, CA

Home run: What the HMO does to hospitalized patients
Shashi K. Agarwal, MD, Orange, NJ

Outfielder positioning: Junior resident in the operating room
S. D. Madduri, MD, Poplar Bluff, MO

Illegal substitution: Generic equivalent disallowed
Hugh H. Wang, MD, Concord, CA

Intentional walk: Physical therapist's procedure
Richard A. Mahrer, MD, San Jose, CA

Buzzer beater: Discharging a patient before the HMO utilization rep has a chance to call you
Arthur E. LaMontagne, Jr., MD, Manchester, CT

Sacrifice fly: Rapid trouser-removal technique in the ER
Melvin J. Breite, MD, Bayside, NY

Base on balls: Sodium hydroxide burn on the scrotum
Gerald Harris, MD, San Francisco, CA

Triple play: HMO decision affecting doctor, hospital, and patient
Joseph B. Szgalsky, MD, Woodbury, NJ

Standing eight count: Number of months waiting for insurers' reimbursement
Daniel J. Colombi, MD, Haddonfield, NJ

Free throws: insurance companies' ability to deselect "providers" without cause.
Gary M. Gorlick, MD, Los Angeles, CA

Loading the bases: Bicarbonate by IV push
Richard H. Dermody, MD, Breese, IL

NOTABLE NEWS

ASSIGNMENT:

Imagine a singing telegram at your door delivered by a uniformed bearer of significant news.

EXAMPLES:

This happy news is overdue
You're targeted for chart review.

To sing you this we're more than proud
Your surgeon's fee is disallowed.

For audit, bring all records soon
The IRS has sent this tune.

ENTRIES:

Bad news by twos just entered your foyer
Your exes are here, and each with a lawyer.

James F. Gardner, MD, San Antonio, TX

Greetings from your HMO
We have your patients, so you can go.

B. L. Weeks, DO, Edmond, OK

Your financial planner wishes you good health
He's landed in Barbados with all your wealth.

Ronald P. Olah, MD, Pasadena, CA

My jingle is short
You're going to court.

Daniel J. Colombi, MD, Haddonfield, NJ

We hope this line gives you a laugh
Your charts are late; you're off the staff.

Allan L. Goldman, MD, Raleigh, NC

Delinquent charts have earned you fame
National Data Bank now carries your name.

Tejinder S. Sandhu, MD, Sanger, CA

The medical review board is sorry to say
We've revoked your license, but have a nice day.

R. Schlein, MD, Richmond, VA

Who's the fairest of them all?
'Tisn't you, so you're on call.

Allan R. LaReau, MD, Portage, MI

Forget about that great vacation
We've just decreased your capitation.

Mona J. Shapiro, Branchburg, VA

Who could possibly ever have guessed?
Your Lexus is being repossessed.

Robert R. Jones, MD, Nevada, MO

Your medical society thinks you're very
Capable—now you're secretary!

R. C. Whitesitt, MD, Helena, MT

Salutations and congratulations
You've joined our HMO and now have 94,564 new patients.

Gary M. Gorlick, MD, Los Angeles, CA

About your patients, Bill and Mary
Their scrips are not on formulary.

Thomas F. Mertins, MD, Warsaw, IN

Your partner left without a fight
You're now on call most every night.

Mark Weinreb, MD, Westminster, MA

Call your lawyer and banker, too
Another patient is suing you.

Alex St. Onge, Brookline, MA

Your skillfully fashioned mammary peaks
Have sadly sprung unsightly leaks.

Joseph F. J. Curi, MD, Torrington, CT

Try to smile from ear to ear
A *60 Minutes* crew is here.

Marilyn B. Price, RN, Gonzales, TX

That pension fund manager you hired last fall
His picture went up—on the post office wall.

Jonathan Ehrlich, MD, Atlanta, GA

The call was from the OR
Your case for eight is now at four.

Neal Green, MD, Corsicana, TX

MATING SEASON

ASSIGNMENT:

Compose a medical person's companion-seeking ad, as in the personals.

EXAMPLES:

Sleep lab technician, a pillow of the community, seeks to REMedy loneliness.

Blood bank supervisor wishes to form lifelong agglutination with someone of sanguine disposition and type A (B, O, AB) personality.

Endocrinologist with a fine sense of humor desires hormonic relationship. Send photo and corticosteroid titer.

ENTRIES:

Ophthalmologist SEEks focus with EYEdeal partner for 20/20 farsighted relationship.

Morey Filler, MD, San Francisco, CA

Pathologist desires conversation, relationship. Not picky, just want a companion who is alive.

Kathy Waller, MD, Fort Collins, CO

High-powered pathologist seeks cellmate for benign relationship with rapid growth potential, nonsmoking specimens only. Must enjoy fixing things and seeing the cytes. Should be a blast. Send color slides to . . .

James F. Gardner, MD, San Antonio, TX

Holistic herbalist looking for nature-loving partner to smell the roses, decoct their essence, and infuse them into the body, mind, and spirit!

Samuel M. Grief, MD, Portsmouth, NH

Hospital chaplain who practices what he preaches, experienced, wishes a lady of clean body, clean thoughts. Will take either one.

Joel T. Appleton, MD, Abilene, TX

Podiatrist seeks solemate. Please, no corny jokesters.

Stephen Lieberman, MD, Clackamas, OR

Microscopist who understands the Big Picture, desires to begin a nuclear family with one who appreciates the little things in life.

Carlyn M. Kline, MD, St. Joseph, MO

Primary care, managed-care physician seeking capitating (and captivating) companion—no authorization required.

Roland P. Olah, MD, Pasadena, CA

Infectious disease specialist desires to reach out and touch someone. Please submit photo, résumé of most recent STD titers, and glove size.

Jerome M. Eder, MD, Agoura, CA

Anesthesiologist: N_2Orgies; can go ether way; let's have a gas together.

B. L. Weeks, DO, Edmond, OK

Toxicologist who takes needling easily, good at hashing out differences, seeks nonvein woman who gets a bhang out of mindless activities like nosing through junk stores.

Douglas Ackerman, MD, Clackamas, OR

Stable psychiatrist interested in meeting someone ready to be committed.

Hugh H. Wang, MD, Concord, CA

Music-loving gastroenterologist wishes to intussuscept with potential partner to share life's borborygmi.

Alan R. Seplowitz, MD, New York, NY

Laryngoscopic surgeon thinking remotely of relationship that can be opened into full-bodied exploration if indicated. Videos a necessity.

Melvin J. Breite, MD, Bayside, NY

Neurologist seeks man who, at one stroke, possesses brains and nerve, and is well-coordinated and rich. Endorphins need not apply. Will take ataxia to meet you for a marche a petit pas on the hippocampus.

Paul B. Ross, MD, Great Neck, NY

TO THE LETTER

ASSIGNMENT:
Subtract a letter from a well-known non-English term, deriving a medical interpretation therefrom.

EXAMPLES:
Wetschmerz: Diaper rash
Mano a ano: Prostate examination
Amicus uriae: A friendly nephrologist
Pro bono pubico: Motto of urological association

ENTRIES:
Ecce HMO: Behold the manacles.

Raymond J. Gaspari, MD, Bountiful, UT

Faux pas: A welcomed paternity test result

Michael B. Curi, Farmington, CT

Ma de mer: Delivery at sea

David A. Kline, MD, Los Angeles, CA

Auf widersehen: Now you will have a much bigger visual field.

Meyer B. Hodes, MD, East Rockaway, NY

Corpus electi: A deceased politician

Vincent L. Keipper, MD, Concord, NC

C'est la ie: Pulmonologist eliciting an egophony

David M. Bergdahl, MD, Fresno, CA

Much cojones: Advanced bilateral hydrocele

Julio C. Novoa, MD, Perrry Hall, MD

Kemo abe: Native American drug therapy for the 16th president

Joseph F. J. Curi, MD, Torrington, CT

Vive le oi: The bane of pain centers

Daniel J. Colombi, MD, Haddonfield, NJ

Sin qua non: Sending a patient to a non-HMO contract facility
Hugh H. Wang, MD, Concord, CA

Que sera era: Huge lab mistake
Irving Thorne, MD, Minneapolis, MN

Allegro no troppo: A fast-acting generic antidepressant
A. Zambra, MD, Houston, TX

"L'Arsellaise": Anthem for colonoscopists
Mark M. Benkel, MD, Brooklyn, NY

Ax vobiscum: Motto of HMO utilization panel.
Edward M. Sessa, MD, Schenectady, NY

¿No es erdad?: We'll need DNA testing
Carlyn M. Kline, MD, St. Joseph, MO

Oi polloi: Pain caused by injuries common to the masses
A. Schlein, Richmond, VA

Ubris: Do-it-yourself circumcision
Dan Steinbrocker, Los Angeles, CA

Fat accompli: Dietitian
Daniel C. Ginsberg, MD, Gig Harbor, WA

Zitgeist: The teenage years
Howard F. Heller, MD, Montlake Terrace, WA

Stabat mate: Domestic violence
Melvin J. Breite, MD, Bayside, NY

Magnum pus: Infected gunshot wound
Yvonne Lyles, MD, Beaverton OR

Erra incognita: Why I didn't pass my boards?
Ron Hall, MD, Fort Wayne, IN

APPLIED QUOTATIONS

ASSIGNMENT:

Explain a well-known military or political quotation using a medical scenario.

EXAMPLES:

"I shall return."—Lab technician contemplating another spin of the centrifuge

"I do not choose to run." Patient requesting a slowdown of the treadmill

"It's morning in America." Phlebotomist awakening the ward for 5:00 AM venepunctures

"It's the economy, stupid." HMO director setting down a minimal hospitalization policy to the board

ENTRIES:

"War is hell."—Doctor leaving a meeting with HMO reps

> Jeffery J. Rabinovitz, MD, Placerville, CA

"Veni, vidi, vici."—Varicose vein surgeon's operative note

> Bernadine Z. Paulshock, MD, Wilmington, DE

"Fifty-four forty or fight."—Cardiac surgeon discussing fee with HMO clerk

> Douglas Ackerman, MD, Clackamas, OR

"They shall not pass."—Urologist viewing an X-ray of two kidney stones

> Leonard Schreier, MD, Bloomfield Hills, MI

"Après nous le déluge."—Nurse instilling IV lasix

> Dr. Dean Lasseter, Warsaw, IN

"Go for broke."—HMO reimbursement plan

> Daniel J. Colombi, MD, Haddonfield, NJ

"That's voodoo economics."—The collective thought of physicians on the subject of capitation

> Neal Green, MD, Corsicana, TX

"I don't care how you do it; you must sink the Bismarck."—Nutritionist counseling patient with anorexia

Anita Grinis, Kenosha, WI

"I feel your pain"—Marginal anesthesiologist

Russell J. Cox, MD, Gastonia, NC

"I will go to Korea."—Medical resident fulfills his military obligation to Berry Plan

Paul Ross, Great Neck, NY

Similarly, Melvin J. Breite, MD, Bayside, NY

"Let them eat cake."—Hospital dietitians' strike placard

Arthur E. LaMontagne, Jr., MD, Manchester, CT

". . . ask not what your country can do for you . . ."—Doctor informing patient he does not accept Medicare assignments

Luann Woods, DO, Ada, OK

"Follow me, men."—The cardiac rehabilitation leader in shorts

Gary M. Gorlick, MD, Los Angeles, CA

"Tear down that wall."—Physician expanding his practice

R. Schlein, MD, Richmond, VA

". . . a date which will live in infamy"—Start-up of the first HMO

Floyd T. Nasuti, MD, Philadelphia, PA

Similarly, Herbert Gersh, MD, Treaure Island, FL

". . . that's one small step for a man . . ."—Neurologist on Parkinsonian shuffle

Katie Norton, MD, Omaha, NE

"Let's move on."—HMO patient being informed that his authorized hospital stay has been canceled

Thomas Y. Fung, MD, Hayward, CA

"Fourscore and seven years . . ."—HMO medical director explaining time needed for procedure approval

Joseph B. Szgalsky, MD, Woodbury, NJ

"I come here tonight with a heavy heart."—Transplant surgeon bearing donor heart with unexpected amyloidosis

Gene Westveer, MD, Zeeland, MI

THE NAME GAME

ASSIGNMENT:
Name a well-known nonfictional, contemporary person whose name is applicable to a medical pursuit.

EXAMPLES:
Gary Hart: Cardiologist
Oral Roberts: Dentist
John McCain: Physical therapist
I. M. Pei: Medical insurer's reimbursement officer

ENTRIES:
Tupac: Pulmonologist

> Joseph F. J. Curi, MD, Torrington, CT

Amelia Earhart: Otolaryngologist and cardiologist

> L. H. Schilling, MD, Fresno, CA

Mark McGwire: Interventional radiologist

> John S. Fox, MD, Richland, WA
> Similarly, Charles G. Eschenburg, MD, Boynton Beach, FL

Drew Bledsoe: Inept phlebotomist

> Mackenzie Smith, MD, Mercer Island, WA
> Similarly, Arthur E. LaMontagne, Jr., MD, Manchester, CT

Nora Ephron (N. Ephron): Nephrologist

> Michael Ichniowski, MD, Lutherville, MD

Mary Chapin-Carpenter: Double boarded-dermatology, orthopedics

> Kathy Waller, MD, Fort Collins, CO

Slim Pickens: Dietitian

> Wendy Sweeney, Chula Vista, CA

Norman Schwartzkopf: Dermatologist
Douglas Ackerman, MD, Clackamas, OR

(Any) Rockefeller: Lithotripsy specialist
Robert Resnick, MD, Forest Hills, NY

The Smothers Brothers: Respiratory therapists
R. Schlein, MD, Richmond, VA

David Hyde Pierce: Acupuncturist
Carol Scharf, Hamden, CT

Tipper Gore: Medical examiner
Shirley Press, MD, Miami Beach, FL

Phil Gramm: Pharmacist
Russell J. Cox, MD, Gastonia, NC

Sarah Bernhardt: Specialist in reflux esophagitis
Daniel J. Colombi, MD, Haddonfield, NJ

Chubby Checker: Bariatrician
Nicholas M. Cifelli, Jr., MD, Fort Myers, FL

Werner Erhard: Respiratory therapist
Paul B. Ross, MD, Great Neck, NY

Danny Glover: Proctologist
L. Robert Rubin, MD, Danbury, CT

Engelbert Humperdinck: Peyronie's disease specialist
Richard K. Crissman, MD, Wyoming, MI

Kevin Spacey: Anesthesiologist
Amy Porter, MD, La Cañada, CA

Peter Sellers: Penile implant salesman
Daniel P. Sporn, MD, Athens, PA

Al Hirt: Pain management specialist

Gerry Farmer, MD, LaGrange, GA

Whoopie Goldberg: ID physician with special interest in pertussis

Hugh H. Wang, MD, Concord, CA

Malcolm X: Radiologist

Julio Novoa, MD, Perry Hall, Lutherville, MD

David Letterman: Optometrist

Lenard Silverman, MD, Alpharetta, GA

Elizabeth Dole: Social worker

Thomas R. White, MD, St. Petersburg, FL

Ravi Shankar: Sexually transmitted disease specialist

Alan L. Goldman, MD, Raleigh, NC

DUPLEX

ASSIGNMENT:
Since some doctors have dual jobs, document this in a terse rhyme, suitable for letterhead.

EXAMPLES:
Pathologist: Lab and slab
Urologist: Circ and perc
Neurosurgeon: Pain and brain

ENTRIES:
Neonatal cardiologist: Qs and blues

> Neal Green, MD, Corsicana, TX

Allergist: Mast and rast

> Arthur N. Feinberg, MD, Kalamazoo, MI

Pathologist: Issues and tissues

> Meyer B. Hodes, MD, East Rockaway, NY

Cardiologist: Tracings and pacings

> Michael Ichniowski, MD, Lutherville, MD

Oncologist: Hemo and chemo

> Barni Schlein, Richmond, VA

Dermatologist: Laser and razor

> Sandra S. Mamis, Poughkeepsie, NY
> Similarly, Robert Resnick, MD, Forest Hills, NY

Pediatrician: Germs and worms

> Myron Siner, MD, Wellesley, MA

OB-GYN: Slap and Pap

> David A., Kline, MD, Los Angeles, CA

Gastroenterologist: Cope and scope

Rajender K. Arora, MD, Orange, NJ

Mexican urologist: Stones and cojones

Robert Ettlinger, MD, Millersburg, PA

Dermatologist: Dry it and fry it

Edward M. Thompson, MD, Clearwater, FL

Otolaryngologist: Rhinos and sinus

Mona Shapiro, Stockton, NJ

Alternative medicine man: Gink and zinc

Joseph F. J. Curi, MD, Torrington, CT

Ophthalmologist: Vision and incision

Melvin J. Breite, MD, Bayside, NY; R. Schlein, Richmond, VA

Pulmonologist: Honk and bronch

David Felker, MD, Delray Beach, FL

Family practitioner: From burp to TURP

Thomas J. Durkin, Jr., MD, Fort Washington, PA

HMO CEO: Denial and decrial

David Perkins, MD, Blue Bell, PA

Neurologist: Seizures and amnesias

Irving Thorne, MD, Minneapolis, MN

SIGN LANGUAGE

ASSIGNMENT:
In the fashion of football referees, contrive an arcane signal to communicate a medical event.

EXAMPLES:
Right hand taps left wrist, elbow, both knees, and right shoulder. (The Joint Commission is about to arrive.)

Left leg is fixed; right leg swings in pendulum fashion. (The hospital building fund kickoff is at hand.)

A handkerchief is tossed to the floor, followed by several taps to the side of the nose. (An allergy patient is in the waiting room.)

ENTRIES:
Right arm raised straight overhead; both arms raised and crossed behind head; left arm raised straight overhead twice. (IX, I, I, or "Call 911")

Jerome M. Eder, MD, West Hills, CA

Right hand to forehead, then sternum, then left shoulder and right shoulder; followed by clasping both hands in front of sternal midline. (Registered letter from a plaintiff's attorney is imminent.)

Daniel J. Colombi, MD, Haddonfield, NJ

Fist closed, thumb extended downward. (Response of managed care to authorization request)

Floyd T. Nasuti, MD, Philadelphia, PA

Both hands thrust upward, followed by total body supination. (Final surrender to the new insurance clerk)

Joel T. Appleton, MD, Abilene, TX

3-0 silk thrown at circulator; 1-0 silk thrown at scrub nurse; 2-0 nylon thrown at anesthetist. (Surgeon needs a 2-0 silk suture.)

Irving Thorne, MD, Minneapolis, MN

Tap wristwatch twice; point one fully extended arm straight up; point the other straight down. (Chief resident reminds surgical intern that the operation will begin when the big hand is on the 12 and the little hand is on the 6.)

Joseph F. J. Curi, MD, Torrington, CT

Both hands placed successively over ears, eyes, mouth; then slash sign across neck. (No more phone calls.)

Russell J. Cox, MD, Gastonia, NC

Physician spins around while pointing to his mouth with one hand and to an infant with the other. (Give this baby the oral rotavirus vaccine.)

Alan L. Goldman, MD, Raleigh, NC

Pull hair, then stretch out arms. (The harried mother with the bratty triplets has arrived.)

Charles G. Eschenburg, MD, Boynton Beach, FL

Index finger in each ear; two or three kicks with either foot; then nostrils pinched shut. (A screaming kicker with a dirty diaper in the examining room)

G. J. Billmeier, Jr., MD, Memphis, TN

Stick pinkies in ears. (Set up ear-cleaning equipment.) Stick fingers in ears (Turn down radio.) Stick thumbs in ears. (Heartfelt message to HMO.)

Melvin J. Breite, MD, Bayside, NY

A yellow card waved frantically. (Bilirubin level is out of bounds.)

C. M. McKenzie, Jr., MD, Columbia, SC

A TAXING ASSIGNMENT

ASSIGNMENT:
In a space at the end of a fictional tax form, have your say in the form of a one-line remark.

EXAMPLES:
This is epistaxis: paying through the nose.
End stage phlebotomy!
The rhythm is bad enough, but the rate . . . !

ENTRIES:
My dues unto Caesar—sans anesthesia
> Tejinder S. Sandhu, MD, Sanger, CA

Golytely on me—I'm all cleaned out now!
> Susan L. Auffinger, MD, Clemmons, CA

Labor and Delivery
> Robert O. Wilson, MD, Fresno, CA

You and my HMO got the uranium mine; I got the shaft.
> Daniel J. Colombi, MD, Haddonfield, NJ

The tap is now dry.
> Joanne M. Demas, MD, Columbus, OH

Immune-deficient monetary incontinence!
> Meyer B. Hodes, MD, East Rockaway, NY

I guess urologists aren't the only ones who can get blood from a stone.
> Herbert Gersh, MD, Treasure Island, FL

. . . made me deliver via vaccum extraction, plus the Credé maneuver.
> Julio Novoa, MD, Perry Hall, MD; Similarly,
> David A. Kline, MD, Los Angeles, CA

Break out the EMLA: This is painful!

Allan R. LaReau, MD, Vicksburg, MI

After this catharsis, I remain financially cachectic.

Joseph F. J. Curi, MD, Torrington, CT

Punch biopsy of the wallet.

Russell J. Cox, MD, Gastonia, NC

You IRS types could use an orthodontist for your big overbite.

Leonard W. Rozin, MD, Oklahoma City, OK

Status epilepticus: one seizure after another.

Michael Curi, Farmington, CT

My account has been cleaned out via a financial purgative.

Alan L. Goldman, MD, Raleigh, NC

If you like 38% of my income so much, why did you cut my Medicare fees?

Melvin J. Breite, MD, Bayside, NY

Monetopenia . . . exsanguination.

S. D., Madduri, MD, Poplar Bluff, MO

You take it off one's hide better than a laser does tattoos.

Jane Niese, RN, Findlay, OH

You have made me into a nonprofit corporation.

R. Schlein, MD, Richmond, VA

Alas, Oh Death—where is thy sting? I'm looking at it.

Stan Hines, MD, Huntsville, TX

GETTING THERE

ASSIGNMENT:
Name a vehicle that leaves little doubt as to what medical facility awaits its passengers.

EXAMPLES:
Nephrology clinic: Dialy-Ride
Infectious disease hospital: The Buggy
ENT clinic: The Eustacian Wagon
Ectopic pregnancy care facility: The Tube

ENTRIES:
Strabismus treatment center: Oculomotorcycle

> Eva Briggs, MD, Marcellus, NY

Geriatric Clinic: Lincoln Incontinental; Cadillac Elderado

> Dave Taube, MD, Oak Harbor, WA

Eye clinic, conjunctivitis division: The Red Eye

> Robert Resnick, MD, Forest Hils, NY

Hematology center: B_{12} Bomber

> Dorrie Christman, MD, Largo, FL

Diabetology OPD: The Sugarland Express

> Daniel J. Colombi, MD, Haddonfield, NJ

Laparoscopy surgery center: The Tro-Car

> Evelyn L. Weissman, MD, Malone, NY

Dementia clinic: Dinghy

> Hugh H. Wang, MD, Concord, CA

Multispecialty clinic: The Omnibus

> Alan L. Goldman, MD, Raleigh, NC

HMO clinic: Managed Caravan

Thomas A. Hopkins, MD, Springfield, MO

Allergy clinic: The Whealbarrow

Charles Webb, MD, Traverse City, MI

Diabetes clinic: The Glucose Transporter

S. Haque, MD, Buffalo, NY

Rehab facility: PT Boat

Mackenzie Smith, MD, Mercer Island, WA

Hematology office: Band Wagon

Floyd T. Nasuti, MD, Philadelphia, PA

Otology OPD: Semicircular Canal Boat

Nicholas M. Cifelli, Jr., MD, North Fort Myers, FL

Russian urology office: Uroflot

Dean Hadley, MD, Paradise, CA

Cardiology center: Paddlewheeler

R. Schlein, MD, Richmond, VA

Amenorrhea clinic: Unicycle

Rudi Kirschner, MD, Phoenix, AZ

Proctology clinic: The Glove Boat

Cynthia and Ronald Barabas, MDs, West
Allenhurst, NJ

Dumping syndrome facility: Rapid Transit

Daniel Schual-Berke, MD, Seattle, WA
Similarly, Paul Van Ausdal, MD,
Yellow Springs, OH

Incontinence clinic: Puddle Jumper

Glenn S. Sherman, MD, Allentown, PA

Hand surgery building: Magic Carpus
>> Gail Cawkwell, MD, Las Vegas, NV

Pulmonary clinic: Monorâle
>> Dr. Martin Lipton, Carmel, NY

Alcoholism clinic: The Wagon
>> Bernadine Z. Paulshock, MD, Wilmington, DE

Depression clinic: The Lift
>> Brett Johnson, MD, Erie, PA

Pain center: Hertz Rent-A-Car
>> Thomas S. Del Giorno, Jr., MD, Philadelphia, PA

Breast augmentation surgicenter: The Front End Loader
>> Carol Ward, MD, Portland, ME

Obesity clinic: One Ton Pickup
>> Russell J. Cox, MD, Gastonia, NC

Neonatology facility: The Cord-o-van
>> Elaine Schwab, Albany, NY

DOLOROUS

ASSIGNMENT:
Match a medical setting with an appropriate word or expression for a bad outcome or situation.

EXAMPLES:
Optical shop—Framed
Fracture clinic—Cast out
Podiatry office—Booted out

ENTRIES:
Managed care office—Decapitated
David M. Pollack, MD, Swarthmore, PA

Two-doctor proctology group—Assassinated
Leon Hodes, MD, East Rockaway, NY

Urology clinic—Rendered intestate
Alan H. Seplowitz, MD, New York, NY

EKG/EEG testing site—Ill at EE's
Morey Filler, MD, San Francisco, CA

Fracture clinic—Castigated
William Zavod, MD, Merion, PA

Impotency clinic—Stiffed
Kathy Waller, MD, Fort Collins, CO

Cryotherapy clinic—Frozen out
Paul A. Rozeboom, MD, Davenport, IA

Ophthalmology office—Stymied
Herbert Gersh, MD, Treasure Island, FL

Plastic surgery clinic—Flat busted

Eva F. Briggs, MD, Marcellus, NY
Similarly, Cathy Dillon, DO, Gibsonia, PA

Anesthesiology office—Down and out

Aaron N. Newberg, MD, Huntingdon Valley, PA

Hematology lab—Double (typed and) crossed

Glenn S. Sherman, MD, Allentown, PA

Urology clinic—Drained

Joel T. Appleton, MD, Abilene, TX

Cardiology clinic—Wolff-Parkinson-white-out

L. Shakerin, MD, Robbinsdale, MN

Infertility clinic—Superseded

Meyer B. Hodes, MD, East Rockaway, NY

Orthopedic clinic—Pinned down and screwed up

Sudhir L. Prabhu, MD, Jacksonville, FL

Pharmacy—Dispensed with

S. A. Hollander and V. Berkovich, MDs,
Lakewood, NJ

Amputation surgicenter—Stumped

Tejinder S. Sandhu, MD, Sanger, CA
Similarly, Carl Sorgen, MD, Poughkeepsie, NY

Outside proctologist's office—Rear-ended

Oscar Venzor, DO, Tampa, FL

Dwarfism endocrinology clinic—Belittled

Joseph F. J. Curi, MD, Torrington, CT

Orthopedic department—Given the cold shoulder

Christopher M. Alinea, MD, New Hartford, NY

Urology office—Given the finger

Stephen E. Halpin, MD, Hannibal, MO

ENT OPD—Croaked

Alan L. Goldman, MD, Raleigh, NC

Mammography office/clinic—Pressed to the limit

Anita Connell, MD, Seattle, WA

Radiology department—Exposed

Patrice Vorwerk, MD, Setauket, NY

Similarly, Ronald P. Olah, MD, Pasadena, CA

Plasmapheresis suite—Washed out

Jan R. J. de Vries, MD, Boswell, PA

GI endoscopy lab—Gutted

Patricia J. Peterson, MD, Longview, WA

ENT clinic—Waxed

Douglas Ackerman, MD, Clackamas, OR

Arthroscopic clinic—Kneedy

Leo Westmoreland, MD, Hammond, LA

IN ITS RIGHTFUL PLACE

ASSIGNMENT:
Link a medical-related group or event to an appropriate venue.

EXAMPLES:
Oral surgery: Boca Grande
Sinusitis group: Carlsbad Caverns
Orthopedists: Wounded Knee
Peptic Ulcer Society: Crater Lake

ENTRIES:
Munchausen Convention: Champaign, IL
E. M. McMahon, MD, Seattle, WA

Hematology group: Santa Fe, NM
Floyd T. Nasuti, MD, Philadelphia, PA

Contraceptive research group: Great Barrier Reef
P. Menon, MD, Mountain View, CA

Vasectomists: Baghdad
Dave Taube, Oak Harbor, WA

Dermatologists: Spotsylvania County, VA
Janet Adams, MD, Silver Spring, MD

Dental Historical Society: Woodbridge, NJ
Glenn S. Sherman, MD, Allentown, PA

Alcoholism Historical Study Society: Lake Mead
Ronald L. Pennington, MD, Newport Beach, CA

Annual Enterovesical Fistulas Conference: Pierre, SD
Roger D. Rosenquist, MD, Portland, OR

Dermatologists' choral group: Singapore
Madeleine Neems, MD, Highland Park, IL

Paget's Disease Society: Marblehead, MA
Meyer B. Hodes, MD, East Rockaway, NY

Depression Treatment Society: Dismal Swamp, VA
Lois A. Miles, MD, Decatur, GA

Monthly Seizure Disorder Meeting: Shaker Village, NH
Anthony Battista, MD, Stewart Manor, NY

HMO Gatekeepers: Grants Pass, OR
Alex Zambra, MD, Houston, TX

Symposium on Cat Scratch Disease: Los Gatos, CA
Luis E. Ruiz, MD, Tehachapi, CA

Central Venous Catheter Course: Newport News, VA
Susan L. Auffinger, MD, Clemmons, NC; Morey
Filler, MD, San Francisco, CA; Margaret M.
Stone, MD, Woodland Hills, CA

HMO Preauthorization Committee: Milidawadawoerzuzizhiqi, Russia
Tejinder S. Sandhu, MD, Sanger, CA

Pediatric Surgery and Vaccine Committees meet concurrently at Cut and Shoot, Texas.
Heather Daniels, MD, Tacoma., WA

Pain control specialists: Aiken, SC
Arnold I. Shatz, MD, Santa Ana, CA

Premature Ejaculation Prevention Group: Rapid City, SD
John J. Swain, MD, Tucson, AZ

Diabetes conference: Sweet Home, OR

Ron Sklar, MD, Portland, OR

Transplant hepatologists: Liverpool

Joseph F. J. Curi, MD, Torrington, CT

Cryptorchidism Society: Bali H'ai

Paul Van Ausdal, MD, Yellow Springs, OH

Conference on Sonography, CT, MRI: Scandinavia

Jonathan Ehrlich, MD, Atlanta, GA

START THE PRESSES

ASSIGNMENT:
Select a well-known play, then spin it into a medical headline.

EXAMPLES:
Inherit the Wind: New Respiratory Therapy Group Takes Over.
The Tempest: Factional Battle Rages As Two Large Hospitals Merge
Tobacco Road: Details of COPD Evolution Bared

ENTRIES:
The Importance of Being Earnest: Gender Surgery is Successful
Joel T. Appleton, MD, Abilene, TX

I Love You, You're Perfect, Now Change: Plastic Surgeon and Psychiatrist to Run Joint Workshop.
Charles G. Eschenburg, MD, Boynton Beach, FL

Barefoot in the Park: Physician Reimbursement Hits an All-Time Low
Daniel J. Colombi, MD, Haddonfield, NJ

The Merchant of Venice: Bloodless Surgery Not Feasible; Court Finds for Patient
Michael R. Popovic, MD, Santa Ana, CA

Candide: Travels of a Yeast
Nicholas M. Cifelli, Jr., MD, North Fort Myers, FL

Salome: John's HMO is capitated
Paul B. Ross, Flushing, NY

The Miracle Worker: Medicare Computers Y2K-Ready
Donna L. Lupski, MD, Berkeley Heights, NJ

Voices in the Dark: Radiologists Are Consulting Today
Floyd T. Nasuti, MD, Philadelphia, PA

Back to Methuselah: New Longevity Advances—Are They Worth It?
Meyer B. Hodes, MD, East Rockaway, NY

Ragtime: Gauze Sponges on Back Order; Severe Shortage Expected
Jonathan S. Ehrlich, MD, Atlanta, GA

Epic Proportions: Urologists Present Their Case of the Month
Bernadine Z. Paulshock, Wilmington, DE

Guys and Dolls: New Medical Specialty Clinic Opens in Las Vegas
Stan Hines, MD, Huntsville, TX

The Happy Journey to Camden and Trenton: New Sedative Safe and Effective for Traveling Children
Russell J. Cox, MD, Gastonia, NC

DOMICILIARY

ASSIGNMENT:
Coin a name for a street or housing project where groups of similar physicians would reside.

EXAMPLES:
Surgeons: Kutting Korners
Obstetricians: Belly Achers
Pulmonologists: Wheezy Street

ENTRIES:
Abdominal surgeons: Ileal Loop

Robert A. Gerber, MD, Sherman Oaks, CA

Psychiatrists: Borderline Development

Vladimir Berkovich, MD and Sharon A.
Hollander, PsyD, Lakewood, NJ

Pathologists: Rue Morgue

Floyd T. Nasuti, MD, Philadelphia, PA

Geriatricians: Withering Heights

R. Schlein, Richmond, VA

Proctologists: Glover's Lane

Charles W. Webb, MD, Traverse City, MI

Neurologists: Hippocampus

Douglas Ackerman, MD, Clackamas, OR

Obstetricians: The Breakwater

Herbert Gersh, MD, Treasure Island, FL

Psychiatrists: Id Row

Daniel J. Colombi, MD, Haddonfield, NJ

Bariatricians: Broadwalk
Joseph F. J. Curi, MD, Torrington, CT

General surgeons: Appy'n Way
David A. Zomick, MD, Bristol, CT

Gastroenterologists: Magenstrasse
Rudi Kirschner, MD, Phoenix, AZ

Adolescent pediatricians: Juvenile Court
John D. Moroney, MD, Tampa, FL

Cardiologists: Atrial Complex
Nirupama Madduri, MD, Huntington, WV

Orthopedists: The Backyard
Grafton C. Fanney, Jr., MD, Euclid, OH

Bariatricians: Fast Lane
Morey Filler, MD, San Francisco, CA

Gastroenterologists: Liver's Lane
Vincent Napoliello, MD, Wayne, NJ

Urologists: The Brownstone
John Knight, MD, Huntsville, TX

Anesthesiologists: Air Way
Deborah Rotenstein, MD, Pittsburgh, PA

Endocrinologists: Sex Drive
Phil Frankenfeld, PhD., Washington, DC

Anesthesiologists: Twilight Zone:
Sudhir K. Prabhu, MD, Jacksonville, FL

Surgeons: Knot Square
Hugh H. Wang, MD, Concord, CA

Cardiology: Bundle Branch Block

R. Patel, MD, Pasadena, TX

Infectious disease specialists: St. D

Dave Taube, Oak Harbor, WA

Urologists: High Rises

Aaron N. Newberg, MD, Huntingdon Valley, PA

Rheumatologists: Rigid Ridge

Kirk R. Hassenmueller, MD, Rockingham, NC

GPs: Family Circle

Paul M. Dichter, DO, Seminole, OK

Hair transplant surgeons: Mane Street

William G. White, MD, Franklin Park, IL

Hematologists: Blood Drive

Victor Tauro, MD, Lanoka Harbor, NJ

CELESTIAL SIGHTS

ASSIGNMENT:
Give an appropriate medically derived name to an area of a yet-to-be-discovered planet.

EXAMPLES:
The Ulceroid Crater
Incontinental Shelf
The Manic Depression

ENTRIES:
Forameno Valley

> R. M. Kniseley, MD, Oak Ridge, TN

The Frozen Section

> Richard A. Mahrer, MD, San Jose, CA

The Morass of Aitchemos

> Meyer B. Hodes, MD, East Rockaway, NY

The Subduranian Desert

> Richard Julius, MD, and Gloria Julius, St. Petersburg, FL

The Sea of Rupture

> Daniel J. Colombi, MD, Haddonfield, NJ

The Estee Elevation

> Alan L. Goldman, MD, Raleigh, NC

Romberg Falls

> Kent J. Lyon, MD, Thibodaux, LA

Anion Gap

> Lyn S. Aye, MD, Jan Jose, CA

The MD-HMO Rift

> Robert R. Jones, MD, Nevada, MO

The Range of Normals

Russell J. Cox, MD, Gastonia, NC

Bipolar Pits and Depressions

Neal Green, MD, Corsicana, TX

Steppes of Care

Ritchie C. Shoemaker, MD, Pokomoke City, MD

The Optic Chasm

Ron Sklar, MD, Portland, OR

The Anal Fissure

Irving Thorne, MD, St. Louis Park, MN

Bipolar Ice Caps

Glenn H. Perelson, MD, Chula Vista, CA

Pox Pit

Bernadine Z. Paulshock, MD, Wilmington, DE

The Cerebral Hemisphere

Paul Johnston, MD, Rice Lake, WI

The Range of Motion

R. Schlein, MD, Richmond, VA

The Emesis Basin

Neal M. Fallis, MD, Westborough, MA

The Semicircular Canals

Floyd T. Nasuti, MD, Philadelphia, PA

The Viagra Erectos

Majer Rosenfeld, MD, Forest Hills, NY

The Acneiform Pits

Frank P. Reynolds, MD, Jacksonville, FL

IMPRECATIONS

ASSIGNMENT:
Think of a withering curse with a medical bent.

EXAMPLES
May all your sigmoidoscopies come semiprepped and distended.
May jaundice and cyanosis color you green.
May all your reimbursements be disallowed.

ENTRIES:
May your bookkeeper quit and join the IRS.
>   Bernadine Z. Paulshock MD, Wilmington, DE

May all your breaks be psychotic.
>   Kathy S. Waller, MD, Fort Collins, CO

May your gluteus get even more maximus.
>   Daniel J. Colombi, MD, Haddonfield, NJ

May all your dictations erase before transcription.
>   W. E. Watkins, MD, Nampa, ID

May the size of your prostate equal that of your ego.
>   Jonathan S. Ehrlich, MD, Atlanta, GA

May the interstate be rerouted past your sleep lab.
>   R. Schlein, MD, Richmond, VA

May all your office staff quit without notice the day before your leave
on vacation.
>   E. Jann Offutt, MD, Worthington, OH

May all your medical waste be thrown into your paper-recycling
bin—five minutes before a surprise OSHA visit.
>   Mona Shapiro, Stockton, NJ

May your hands be in casts when your tinea cruris flares.

David Perkins, MD, St. Davids, PA

May all your VBACs be attorneys.

Morey Filler, MD, San Francisco, CA

May your laparoscope run out of gas in midprocedure.

S. D. Madduri, MD, Poplar Bluff, MO

May all your polyps be sessile.

Herbert Gersh, MD, Treasure, Island, FL

May all your Gomco clamps be too large.

Russell J. Cox, MD, Gastonia, NC

May your TURPs and your bank account be in the red.

Arthur E. LaMontagne, Jr., MD, Manchester, CT

May all your implants be rejected.

Arden Bonebrake, MD, Nebraska City, NE

May your islets of Langerhans desert you at dessert.

Joseph F. J. Curi, MD, Torrington, CT

May your beeper always work.

Alan R. LaReau, MD, Kalamazoo, MI

A halt to your meiosis.

Charles G. Eschenburg, MD, Boynton Beach, FL

May your hair follicles die as your sweat glands multiply.

Joel T. Appleton, MD, Abilene, TX

May your HMO de-capitate you

Michael Ichniowski, MD, Lutherville, MD

May all your authorizations be denied.

Michael Olah, MD, Pasadena, CA

May your radiator melt your sharps container.

Melvin J. Breite, MD, Bayside, NY

May you suffer early climacteric—alcohol-induced and Viagra-resistant.

Richard K. Crissman, MD, Grand Rapids, MI

WORD CONVERSION

ASSIGNMENT:
Select an appropriate medical word and give it a nonmedical meaning.

EXAMPLES:
Lordosis: State of being oversupplied with noblemen
Carbuncle: Small sleeping quarters at the back of a van
Decussation: The process of editing a film to earn it a G-rating.

ENTRIES:
Postmenopause: Rest interval on mail route
Donald J. Mikulak, MD, Denville, NJ

Seroma: What you do after you see Paris
Melvin J. Breite, MD, Bayside, NY

Endorphin: A finalized adoption
Joseph F. J. Curi, MD, Torrington, CT

Sphincter: Designer of ancient Egyptian structures
David Taube, Oak Harbor, WA

Metrorrhagia: Expatriate Indian potentate who haunts the Paris subway system
Lynn Zahner, MD, Lawrenceville, GA

Transverse colon: . .
E. Gallenstein, MD, Cincinnati, OH

Galactase: Certification as a Top Gun pilot of the universe
Robert R. Jones, MD, Nevada, MO

Amenorrhea: Excessive piety
Ivan M. Safonoff, MD, Brooklyn, NY

Blastoma: The definitive book on explosions
Tejinder S. Sandhu, MD, Sanger, CA

Chemotaxis: What the Lone Ranger pays on April 15

Anatoly Belilovsky, Brooklyn, NY

Epilate: Pontius Pilate's Web site

Jonathan Ehrlich, MD, Atlanta, GA

Cauterize: Made successful visual contact

Rajender K. Arora, MD, Orange, NJ

Outliers: A command to eject untruthful persons from the room.

Harry L. Stuber, MD, Cookeville, TN

Herpes: Martha Stewart's vegetables

Bernadine Z. Paulshock, MD, Wilmington, DE

Dura mater: Old college

Robert A. Gerber, MD, Sherman Oaks, CA

Lentigenes: Native beans of Australia

Deborah Lemke, MD, Oshkosh, WI

Endophyte: TKO

Daniel J. Colombi, MD, Haddonfield, NJ

Cardiac thrill: Roller-coaster ride

Joseph Szgalsky, MD, Woodbury, NJ

Winterbottom's Sign: Frostbite involving the buttocks

G. J. Billmeier, MD, Memphis, TN

Furuncle: Your father's brother is the recipient

David Perkins, MD, Blue Bell, PA

Bulimia: A surplus of cattle

Walter S. Mazen, Jr., MD, Chico, CA

Gluteus maximus: Roman centurion (rear guard)

Mackenzie Smith, MD, Mercer Island, WA

GE reflux: Restoring electrical power to an old lightbulb

C. McKenzie, Jr., MD, Columbia, SC

Fibula: A little white lie

Anne Walker, MD, Charlotte, NC

Menopause: Male highway rest areas

A. Zambra, MD, Houston, TX

Carotid: Auto junkyard dealer's child's reply to, "What happened to this car?"

William M. Hardman, MD, Lake Wales, FL

JOX TO DOX

ASSIGNMENT:
Apply the nicknames of current and historic figures to careers in medicine.

EXAMPLES:
Pee Wee Reese: Pediatric urologist
The Splendid Splinter (Ted Williams): Orthopedist
The Yankee Clipper (Joe DiMaggio): New England circumciser

ENTRIES:
William "Dollar Bill" Bradley: Head of HMO

Neil Bellovin, MD, Smithtown, NY

Minnesota Fats: Mayo bariatrician

Richard K. Crissman, MD Grand Rapids, MI

Double X (Jimmy Foxx): Geneticist

Douglas Parry, MD, Richmond Hill, GA

James "Bonecrusher" Smith: Chiropractor

Meyer B. Hodes, MD, East Rockaway, NY

Tug McGraw: Obstetrician

Bernadine Z. Paulshock, MD, Wilmington, DE

Charles "Chief" Bender: Head physical therapist

Daniel J. Colombi, MD, Haddonfield, NJ

Will "The Thrill" Clark: Cardiologist

Anthony R. Russo, MD, Chesapeake, VA

Greg "The Shark" Norman: HMO cost-containment expert

Phil Frankenfeld, PhD, Washington, DC

Dick "Night Train" Lane: Moonlighting ER physician

Ritchie C. Shoemaker, MD, Pocomoke, MD

Anfernes "Penny" Hardaway: HMO medical director
Richard E. Behymer, MD, Sonora, CA

The Big Train (Walter Johnson): Residency director
Dave Taube, Oak Harbor, WA

Slingin' Sammy Baugh: ER doc
Floyd T. Nasuti, MD, Philadelphia, PA

Mr. October (Reggie Jackson): Influenza specialist
Don Chiles, MD, Placentia, CA

Oil Can Boyd: Rheumatologist
Ron Sklar, MD, Portland, OR

The Big Hurt (Frank Thomas): Proctologist
Brett Johnson, Erie, PA

The Steel Curtain (Pittsburgh Steelers): Radiology group
Anatoly Belilovsky, MD, Brooklyn, NY

The Bull (Greg Luzinski): Chairman for HMO claims appeals
Joseph B. Szgalsky, MD, Woodbury, NJ

The Gashouse Gang (St. Louis Cardinals): Anesthesiology group
Alan L. Goldman, MD, Raleigh, NC

William "The Refrigerator" Perry: County coroner
H. C. Kayser, MD, Richland, WA

"Too Tall" Jones: Endocrinologist
Herbert Gersh, MD, Trasure Island, FL,
R. Schlein, MD, Richmond, VA

Elroy "Crazy Legs" Hirsch: Correctional orthopedist
Neal Green, MD, Corsicana, TX

"Stone Cold" Steve Austin: Pathologist

Vincent M. Napoliello, MD, Wayne, NJ

Vernon "Lefty" Gomez, Rollie Fingers, Mike "Pinky" Higgins: Hand surgery group

Richard Julius, MD, and Gloria Julius, EdS, St. Petersburg, FL

THE SKY'S THE LIMIT

ASSIGNMENT:
Apply a medical twist to anything astronomical, with a brief elucidation, if needed.

EXAMPLES:
The Lactic Way
Bipolar ice caps
Veinous
Gemini, the Siamese Twins

ENTRIES:
Pegacyst, the Winged, Cavitied Horse
Vincent Napoliello, MD, Wayne, NJ

Urinary Gravel Belt (asteroids)
Daniel L. Diehl, MD, Willow Street, PA

Hale Bopp's Caudal Appendage
Ivan M. Safonoff, MD, Brooklyn, NY

Kyphosagittarius, the Archer
Melvin J. Breite, MD, Bayside, NY

Corona glandis
David Perkins, MD, St. David's, PA

Mare Fecundatis (vacation spot for barren couples)
MacKenzie Smith, MD, Mercer Island, WA

The Great Androgen Galaxy
Anatoly Belilovsky, MD, Brooklyn, NY

The Lunar Chancroid Craters
Julio Cesar Novoa, MD, Perry Hall, MD

The Diaphragmatic Ring of Saturn
Ed Loman, MD, Albuquerque, NM

Peripheral Pulsar

Daniel J. Colombi, MD, Haddonfield, NJ

O'Rhyne, the Prominent-Nosed Hunter

Hugh H. Wang, MD, Concord, CA

Bursa Major (the great compensator)

Seetha Lath, MD, Arcadia, CA

Mars, the Erythematous Planet

Nicolette Baumgartner, MD, Kalamazoo, MI

The Sagittarius Suture

Russell J. Cox, MD, Gastonia, NC

The Astrocyte Belt

W. E. Watkins, MD, Nampa, ID

Chorion, the Fetal Hunter

Floyd T. Nasuti, MD, Philadelphia, PA

Serous, the Leaky Dog Star

Gloria Julius, St. Petersburg, FL

Canis Major and Canis Minor—large and small dog bites

Bernadine Z. Paulshock, MD, Wilmington, DE

Orion's Belt (site of Orion's Beeper)

Allan R. LaReau, MD, Kalamazoo, MI

Unsubstantia Nigra: Black Hole

Mary Ellen Riegel, MD, Pittsford, NY

Black Hole: HMO Pended Claims Department

Morey Filler, MD, San Francisco, CA

Black Hole: Endoscopic view during a power failure

Joseph F. J. Curi, MD, Torrington, CT

FORMATIVE YEARS

ASSIGNMENT:
Describe a (premedicine) stage in a physician's life, linking it to his/her later career, to wit, I knew him/her when he/she . . . .

EXAMPLES:
. . . was inner ears with a student loan (otologist)
. . . was freelancing (phlebotomist)
. . . had empty coffers (pulmonologist)

ENTRIES:
was a catcher in the rye (rural midwife)
Joseph F. J. Curi, MD, Torrington, CT

was only four, playing [sex therapist]
Melvin J. Breite, MD, Bayside, NY

had no stomach for it [gastroenterologist]
Leland Davis, MD, Santa Rosa, CA

was footloose [podiatrist]
Russell J. Cox, MD, Gastonia, NC

was at zero station [obstetrician]
Neal Green, MD, Corsicana, TX

had no interest in going down the tube [endoscopist]
Richard K. Crissman, MD, Grand Rapids, MI

was nothing to sneeze at [allergist]
Leonard Schreier, MD, Bloomfield Hills, MI

was back in alimentary school [gastroenterologist]
Amy Miller, New Orleans, LA

was but a small pain in the neck [neurosurgeon]
Daniel J. Colombi, MD, Haddonfield, NJ

was still afraid of the dark [radiologist]
>   Floyd T. Nasuti, MD, Philadelphia, PA

was all thumbs [hand surgeon]
>   Mona J. Shapiro, Stockton, NJ

was a budding dilettante [obstetrician]
>   Joseph Grayzel, MD, Englewood, NJ

itched for more [dermatologist]
>   L. Romano Jana, MD, Erie, PA

was overdrawn [hematologist]
>   R. Schlein, MD, Richmond, VA

was only a bit down in the mouth [oral surgeon]
>   Frank P. Reynolds, MD, Jacksonville, FL

was less sanguine [hematologist]
>   Arthur E. LaMontagne, MD, Manchester, CT

he was to die for [pathologist]
>   Alan R. LaReau, MD, Kalamazoo, MI

he could even multiply [fertility specialist]
>   Neal Green, MD, Corsicana, TX

PROVERBIAL SECOND CHANCE

ASSIGNMENT:

Due to loss of all the entries in a previous contest, in which proverbs were to be adapted to medical situations, the invitation is repeated. The examples are the same as before, to wit,

A rolling stone thwarts the lithotripter.

A stitch in time can be hemostatic.

Hyperalimentation is thicker than water.

The underinsured and his money are soon parted.

ENTRIES:

He who grafts last grafts best.

Kathlene S. Waller, MD, Fort Collins, CO

Don't count your residents before they match.

Stanley Hartness, MD, Kociusko, MS

He who hesitates is ready for the urologist.

Anne Waller, MD, Charlotte, NC

Can a man take fire in his bosom and not be monitored?

Meyer B. Hodes, MD, East Rockaway, NY

Too many residents spoil the rounds.

Joseph B. Szgalsky, MD, Woodbury, NJ

It is always darkest before uterine contractions become regular.

Daniel J. Colombi, MD, Haddonfield, NJ

A watched boil never pops.

Phil Frankenfeld, PhD, Washington, DC

What's sauce for the goose is plaque for the coronaries.

Alton R. Prihoda, MD, Baytown, TX

'Tis better to give (blood) than to receive.

Rajender K. Arora, MD, Orange, NJ

The way to a man's heart is through his intercostal spaces.

Alan L. Goldman, MD, Raleigh, NC

The way to a man's heart is through a long catheter.

Julio Novoa, MD, Perry Hall, MD

Physicians who don't take a good history are doomed to repeat it.

Vincent L. Keipper, MD, Concord, NC

The physician who treats himself probably won't collect his co-pay.

Michael Ichniowski, MD, Lutherville, MD

It is better to be silent and be thought a fool than to speak and be sued for malpractice.

W. E. Watkins, MD, Nampa, ID

Dyspareunia is better than no pareunia at all.

Leo Westmoreland, MD, Hammond, LA

Make vitamin D while the sun shines.

Arthur N. Feinberg, MD, Kalamazoo, MI

A garlic a day keeps the doctor at bay.

Richard K. Crissman, MD, Grand Rapids, MI

Spare the rod and spoil the urine culture.

Stanely Hartness, MD, Kosciusko, MS

An apple a day keeps the Go-Litely away.

Neal Green, MD, Corsicana, TX

Still water runs high E. coli counts.

Dan Chiles, MD, Placentia, CA

One in the womb is worth two in the petri dish.

Gedas M. Grinis, MD, Kenosha, WI

Don't put all your ova in one petri dish.

Mona Shapiro, Stockton, NJ

If at first you do recede, try, try Rogaine.

Jason M. Kittler, MD, Pittsfield, MA

Every man has his price unless he's in managed care.

Richard Julius, MD, and Gloria Julius, EdS, St
Petersburg, FL

Do unto HMOs before they do unto you.

Robert Edelman, MD, Garden City, NY

An aspirin a day keeps the invasive cardiologist away.

Anthony Russo, MD, Chesapeake, VA

TOOLING AROUND

ASSIGNMENT:
Select a medical instrument or device and attach thereto a nonmedical definition.

EXAMPLES
Heplock: A wrestling hold
Walking cast: Actors whose bus has broken down
Gigli saw: A humorous adage
Stryker frame: A bowling feat

ENTRIES:
IUD: A dyslexic traffic citation

Daniel J. Colombi, MD, Haddonfield, NJ

Speculum: An adventurous stock market investment program

J. Gopin, MD, Old Bridge, NJ

Metzenbaum: The Wizard of Oz set in Shea Stadium

Irving Thorne, MD, St. Louis Park, MN

Crash cart: An amusement park attraction

Ivan Safonoff, MD, Brooklyn, NY

Central line: A critical segment of the script

Douglas Ackerman, MD, Clackamas, OR

Texas catheter: The Tulsa-Galveston oil pipeline

Anatoly Belilovsky, MD, Brooklyn, NY

Manometer: An instrument to measure virility

Alan L. Goldman, MD, Raleigh, NC

Sonogram: Western Union for the visually impaired

Morey Filler, MD, San Francisco, CA

Rhinoscope: An attachment for an African hunting rifle

Richard K. Crissman, MD, Grand Rapids, MI

DeLee trap: A military maneuver used in the Civil War

Russell J. Cox, MD, Gastonia, NC

IV pole: A long-handled garden tool for trimming vines

Jerome M. Eder, MD, West Hills, CA

Army-Navy retractor: An order to retreat

Hugh H. Wang, MD, Concord, CA

Vacuum extractor: An instrument used to try to get money out of an HMO

Anthony Quartell, MD, Livingston, NJ

Rib spreader: A brush for barbecue sauce

Gloria Perelson, MD, Spring Valley, CA

Pacemaker lead: NASCAR pole position

Anne Walker, MD, Charlotte, NC

Flex sig: Versatile forgery

Yvonne M. Lyles, MD, Aloha, OR

Rongeur: A member of the French park police

Edward L. Spenser, DVM, Salinas, CA

Hemostat: Immediate repair of a hemline

Patricia J. Fogle, DO, Berea, KY

Steri-strip: An exotic dancer

Herbert Gersh, MD, Treasure Island, FL

Scalp monitor: General Custer's worst nightmare

Brett Johnson, MD, Erie, PA

A SPEEDY RECOVERY

ASSIGNMENT:
Devise a get-well card in couplet form, specific to the affliction.

EXAMPLES:
Thou canst not help but better feel
Less thirteen pounds of hydrocele.

Good-bye to the scales at the truck-weighing station
After overdue fundoplication.

Let's drink to the joyous termination
Of your trial suppuration.

ENTRIES:
Once freed fore'er of your gallstones
You'll dine with glee on buttered scones.
Charles W. Webb, MD, Traverse City, MI

Right was left and left was right
Now uncrossed, you've better sight.
Bernadine Z. Paulshock, MD, Wilmington, DE

A toast to your remodeled snout
With artistry in and cartilage out.
Floyd T. Nasuti, MD, Philadelphia, PA

As your I&D heals, there's something to ponder
Does abscess make the heart grow fonder?
Michael Ichniowski, MD, Lutherville, MD

'Tis nothing about which to sneeze
You'll soon be free of Lyme disease.
Alan L. Goldman, MD, Raleigh, NC

We sing your praises on the podium
That you now have a normal sodium.

Arthur N. Feinberg, MD, Kalamazoo, MI

To the team you can return, a
Swimmer relieved of otitis externa.

Stuart M. Copperman, MD, Merrick, NY

Snorts of joy, the end of woes
In that they trimmed your bulbous nose.

Stan Hines, MD, Huntsville, TX

Your discharge and the exit door
Await you, survivor of trichophytobezoar.

Edward M. McMahon, Jr., MD, Seattle, WA

I'm glad your doctor hadn't missed
Your hirsute dentate dermoid cyst.

Mark Wiedemann, MD, Coos Bay, OR

Doped and scoped
Good show—you coped.

Patricia J. Fogle, DO, Berea, KY

You can jump like God intended
Since your bladder was suspended.

Richard K. Crissman, MD, Grand Rapids, MI

To celebrate your lithotripsy
'Tis fair to get a wee bit tipsy.

Russell J. Cox, MD, Gastonia, NC

Blow the trumpets, man the phone
You have passed your kidney stone.

Morey Filler, MD, San Francisco, CA

You'll do a back flip in reaction
To your release from spinal traction.

Frank P. Reynolds, MD, Jacksonville, FL

A diller, a dollar, a badly rent collar
I heard you were better, so give me a holler.

Richard and Gloria Julius, St. Petersburg, FL

Post appendectomy joy abounds
Now that you have bowel sounds.

E. Gallenstein, MD, Cincinnati, OH

It's great you let the docs attack
Your large left common carotid plaque.

Ivan Safonoff, MD, Brooklyn, NY

Here's hoping you made the right decision
To have an adult circumcision.

Samuel R. Oleinick, MD, Tulsa, OK

AUTOMOBILITY

ASSIGNMENT:
Apply a medical twist to a car name and identify the health care professional behind the wheel.

EXAMPLES:
Coupe de bille: Medical insurer
Infini-t: Allergist
Styelark: Opthalmologist

ENTRIES:
Alpha-Beta-Gamma Romeo: Radiologist
> Dein M. Shapiro, MD, Stockton, NJ

Suguru: Professional expert medical witness
> R. G. Flood, MD, San Angelo, TX

Merciless Bends: Physiatrist
> Sree Devi Chandrasekhar, MD, New York, NY

Heavy Cap Price: Capitated HMO exec
> Alton R. Prihoda, MD, Baytown, TX

Gnash Rambler: Orthodontist
> Jerome H. Blumen, MD, Highland Beach, FL

Rales Royce: Pulmonologist
> Kathy Waller, MD, Fort Collins, CO

Jeep Papfinder: Cytotechnologist
> David A. Kline, MD, Los Angeles, CA

Nissan Alzheimer: Gerontologist
> Lanny Freshman, MD, Syracuse, NY

Audi(o): Otologist
> Perry D. Mostov, DO, Worthington, OH

T-Cellica: Hematologist

Jonathan S. Ehrlich, MD, Atlanta, GA

Pintoe: Pediatric surgeon

Jerome M. Eder, MD, Agoura, CA

Austin Healey: Texas pediatrician

Mackenzie Smith, MD, Mercer Island, WA

Dodge Peon: Any resident

Dave Taube, MD, Eugene, OR

Ova Achieva: Reproductive medicine specialist

William G. Cabey, MD, Charlotte, NC

Ford Rongeur: Neurosurgeon

Glenn Perelson, MD, Spring Valley, CA

Bonnevillus: Gastroenterologist

Douglas Ackerman, MD, Clackamas, OR

Benz: Hyperbaric specialist

Matthew Kurlan, D.O., Loveland, OH

Lamborygmi: Gastroenterologist

Allan Plaut, MD, Lawrence, NY

Cut-Lass: Gynecologist

Herbert Gersh, MD, Treasure Island, FL

Cutless: Laparoscopic surgeon

Lisa Fortman, MD, Hinsdale, IL; Stan Paras, MD,
Bedford, NH

Incontinental: Urologist

Alan L. Goldman, MD, Raleigh, NC

Volvolus: General surgeon

Diane L. Fine, MD, and Carl R. Baum, MD,
Woodbridge, CT

Croup de Ville: Pediatrician

> John Mossman, MD, Albuquerque, NM

Saaaahb: Otolaryngologist

> Jay D. Smith, MD, West Hartford, CT

Grand (I) Am: Surgeon

> Julia Kurlan, MD, Loveland, OH

Le Barren: Fertility specialist:

> Meyer B. Hodes, MD, East Rockaway, NY

Gland Rover: Endocrinologist

> James D. Moore, Jr., MD, Abingdon, VA;
> Jonathan S. Ehrlich, MD, Atlanta, GA

WITSENDER'S BRAIN

ASSIGNMENT:
Devise and describe a condition peculiar to a specific occupation or activity, along the order of Housemaid's knee or Swimmer's ear.

EXAMPLES:
Bouncer's toe: Pain incurred when a kick misses the ejectee and strikes the door frame

Crapshooter's wrist: Carpalgia from repetitive die-casting motions

Bowman's arm: Welt on an archer's forearm from repeated bowstring strikes

ENTRIES:
Backstroker's knob: A lump on the top of the head from smashing into the end of the pool

Alan L. Goldman, MD, Raleigh, NC

Internist's inertia: A rare condition occurring when quality assurance and utilization review reach perfect equilibrium, resulting in paralytic indecision

Patricia Barwig, MD, Wauwatosa, WI

Political pundit's mouth: Oral tinea pedis

Ivan Safonoff, MD, Brooklyn, NY

Congressman's anosmia: The inability to smell tainted contributions

Ralph M. Kniseley, MD, Oak Ridge, TN

Caber tosser's prolapse: Self-explanatory

Russell J. Cox, MD, Gastonia, NC

Dribbler's foot: Wet sneaker dermatitis

Glenn P. Lambert, MD, Flemington, NJ

Fund-raiser's palm: Contact dermatitis from excessive greasing; may be complicated by handshakes

Robert M. Goldberg, MD, New York, NY

Stock-car racer's tattoo: A permanent imprint across the chest caused by tight seat belts.

Stan Hines, MD, Huntsville, TX

Thumb planus: Deformity from giving too many injections

Rudi Kirschner, MD, Phoenix, AZ

Mailman's ankle: Depressed macular skin markings in opposing canine dentiform distribution located below the Support-hose tan line

Alan R. Prihoda, MD, Baytown, TX

Pizzamaker's palm: Numbness from excessive pounding of the dough

V. Napoliello, MD, Wayne, NJ

Mall foot: Pedal swelling due to all-day walking through a shopping center

Paul Feldheim, MD, Ventura, CA

Cop's lick spot: Perioral irritation in doughnut-munching policemen

Daniel J. Colombi, MD, Haddonfield, NJ

Yodeler's larynx: Vocal cord strain from trying to make oneself heard throughout the Alps

Gene Westveer, MD, Zeeland, MI

Student's palm: Hand callus from repetitive slapping of the Snooze button on the alarm

Aletha Oglesby, MD, Tulsa, OK

Claustro-toe-bia: Queasy feeling experienced by toes when squeezed into a too-small shoe

Miles Klein, MD, Frisco, TX

Surgeon's elbow: Extensor tendonitis from improper technique in throwing instruments

William G. White, MD, Franklin Park, IL

YOU'VE GOT MAIL

ASSIGNMENT:
Create an e-mail address appropriate to someone laboring in the health care industry.

EXAMPLES:
Otolaryngologist: sayahsayah@nares.com
Two-specialty practitioner: board@certcert.combo
Family practitioner: onlyexneonates@all.com

ENTRIES:
Dermatologist: *gotdotcome@got.com*

Melvin J. Breite, MD, Bayside, NY

Five-man cardiology group: *vtach@qrscomplex.com*

S. D. Madduri, MD, Poplar Bluff, MO

Gastroenterologist: *end2end@last.com*

Clara M. Cubberly, RN, Biloxi, MS

Obstetrician-gynecologist: *bcp4me@0kids.com*

Morey Filler, MD, San Francisco, CA

Sex therapist: *yahoo@org.org.org*

Leland G. Whitson, MD, Manhattan Beach, CA

Urologist: *viagradoc@hotmale.com*

Jorge Alexander Perez, MD, Fort Lauderdale, FL

Bipolar depression psychiatrist: *Undivided@tension.com*

Janice Stikman, Peterboro, NH

Anesthesiologist: *URoutNback@gas.com*

James J. Smith, MD, Gilbert, AZ

Ophthalmologist: *20/20@sight.com*

Deborah Lemke, MD, Oshkosh, WI

Pain management specialist: *ouchless@hurtlink.com*

Susan L. Auffinger, MD, Clemmons, NC

HMO client services: *nohelp@all.com*

C. Daniel Allen, MD, Atlanta, GA

General surgeon: *tocutistocure@OR.com*

James M. Friedman, MD, Fort Worth, TX

Physiatrist: *xrsii@therapy.com*

Bernadine Z. Paulshock, MD, Wilmington, DE

Your local government STD clinic: *thecure@pubichealth.*

Mary A. Manton, MD, Storrs, CT

Urgent care physician: *walkin@anytime.com*

Ran Jia, MD, Houston, TX

Gatekeeper: *work24/7@HMO.com*

Abigail Hagler, MD, Yuma, AZ

Urologist: *2PEZCGU@AOL.com*

George Jones, MD, Plainfield, IL

HMO claims department: *denied@coldhearted.outofnet*

Russell J. Cox, MD, Gastonia, NC

Physical therapist: *ucandoitucandoit@PT.com*

Richard Julius, MD, and Gloria Julius

Urologist: *Uromed@P.ALOT.com*

Arthur E. LaMontagne, Jr., MD, Manchester, CT

Diabetologist: *sugartosex@glands.com*

Govindan P. Nair, MD, St. Petersburg, FL

Acupuncturist: *nopainnogain@pokemon.com*

Hugh H. Wang, MD, Concord, CA

Infectious disease specialist: *poxtoxcox@germs.com*

Joseph F. J. Curi, MD, Torrington, CT

Cardiologist: *Gotrhythm?@doubleclick.com*

Thuan L. Tran, MD, Claremont, CA

THE BIG DE

ASSIGNMENT:
Choose a medical word beginning with "De" and give it an imaginative definition.

EXAMPLES:
Decussation: Process of removing someone's tendency to swear
Decorticate: To remove from a courtroom or to disqualify from a tennis match
Dehiscence: Surgery to mute a snake
Detoxify: To silence a clock

ENTRIES:
Decay: To leave the island

Russell J. Cox, MD, Gastonia, NC

Deionization: Psychotherapy to reduce egocentricity

Alfred R. D'Angelo, DO, Ormond Beach, FL

Decubitus: Museum curator who removes all works by Broque, Léger, and Gris

Harry W. Eichenbaum, MD, St. Petersburg, FL

Descending colon: A typo

Daniel J. Colombi, MD, Haddonfield, NJ

Detubate: To rearrange a musical piece for a French horn

Bernadine Z. Paulshock, MD, Wilmington, DE

Deceased: Damaged condition of a typewriter with unresponsive *c* or *d* key

Lana L. Jeng, MD, Arvada, CO

Deganglionate: To break up a troublesome pride of large wild cats

Diana Soares, CMA, Fall River, MA
Similarly, Thuan L. Tran, MD, Claremont, CA

Delirium: State of having one's pocket picked in Italy

> Thomas R. White, MD, St. Petersburg, FL
> Similarly, Brian W. Donnelly, MD, Pittsburgh, PA

Defoliation: Catheter removal

> Neal Green, MD, Corsicana, TX
> Floyd T. Nasuti, MD, Philadelphia

Desiccation: Removing your pit bull from your neighbor's leg

> Steven Block, MD, Lansdale, PA
> Similarly, Hugh H. Wang, MD, Concord, CA

Degustation: Wind abatement

> Kathy Waller, MD, Fort Collins, CO

Dextrosuria: Right-sided micturitional deviation

> Cash Dubigg, MD, Mesilla Park, NM

Depigmentation: Porcine thought processes

> Douglas Ackerman, MD, Clackamas, OR

Detumescence: Grave robbery

> David Rankin, DO, Winchester, VA

Deliver: Hepatectomize

> Seetha Lath, MD, Arcadia, CA

Detumescence: Process of ventilating a mausoleum

> Robert R. Jones, MD, Nevada, MO

Decubitus: A cure of crap-shooting

> Robert E. Resnick, MD, Oceanside, NY

Depigmentation: The first step to becoming a kosher butcher

> Arthur N. Feinberg, MD, Kalamazoo, MI

Debridgement: Cessation of a card game

Joel T. Appleton, MD, Abilene, TX

Desire: To castrate

Vincent L. Keipper, MD, Concord, NC

DOMICILIARY PROCESS

ASSIGNMENT:
Give an appropriate name to a hotel that houses waiting patients for specific procedures.

EXAMPLES:
Ulcer therapy: The Walled-off Gastoria
Urological surgery: Edgewater
Orthopedics: The Wellsprung Arms
Knee replacement: The Olimpic
Hand surgery: The Palmer House
Allergy: The Four Sneezins

ENTRIES:
Chiropractic: The Outback Inn
Stephen Lieberman, MD, Clackamas, OR

Carpal tunnel syndrome in Moscow: Intowrist
Anatoly Belilovsky, MD, Brooklyn, NY

Psychiatry, HMO-style: The Four Sessions
Morey Filler, MD, San Francisco, CA

Sleep disorders: The Apnean Way Hotel
Richard K. Crissman, MD, Grand Rapids, MI

ENT disorders: The Snoutrigger
Douglas Ackerman, MD, Clackamas, OR

Colonoscopies: The Upham
William V. Adler, MD, Downey, CA

Proctology: The Inn of the Sitz Happiness
Stanley Rogers, DO, Oklahoma City, OK

Hemorrhoids: The Tush Mahal
Melvin J. Breite, MD, Bayside, NY

Psychiatry: Waldorf Hysteria

Floyd T. Nasuti, MD, Philadelphia, PA

Otolaryngology: Caesar's Palate

George P. Bunch, MD, Las Vegas, NM

Venereology: Chancre-La

Stephen L. Kaufman, MD, San Francisco, CA

Dog-bite victims: Motel Sics

Anne E. Walker, MD, Charlotte, NC

Drug rehab for physicians: The Narc Hopkins

Neal Green, MD, Corsicana, TX

Pre-circumcision: The Corona Del Mar

Eric Strauss, MD, Palo Alto, CA

Head injuries: CATskills Resort

Dave Taube, MD, Eugene, OR

Obsessive-compulsive HMO directors: House of Ill Compute

Dein M. Shapiro, MD, Stockton, NJ

Women's intestinal diseases: The Gallorrhea

Mackenzie Smith, MD, Mercer Island, WA

Orthopedics: The Breakers

Thomas R. White, MD, St. Petersburg, FL

Epilepsy: Seizer's Palace

Arthur N. Feinberg, MD, Kalamazoo, MI

Mammoplasty (augmentation): The Builtmore

Bernadine Z. Paulshock, MD, Wilmington, DE

Hematologist: The Plazma

Bruce Ellsweig, MD, Zionsville, PA

Adolescent psychiatry: Youth Hostile
> Mona Shapiro, Stockton, NJ

Neurosurgery: The Fontanelle Blew
> Daniel J. Colombi, MD, Haddonfield, NJ

Proctological surgery: Rump Palace
> Paul B. Ross, MD, Great Neck, NY

Marriage counseling: Marrialot Hotels
> Russell J. Cox, MD, Gastonia, NC

Neurology: Daze Inn
> Louis J. Marchetti, MD, Vass, NC
> Brian W. Donnelly, MD, Pittsburgh, PA

TAKE A HAIKU

ASSIGNMENT:
Using the Haiku verse form, do a modest medical scenario.

EXAMPLES:
Gatekeeper's office
Smallish time for each patient
King of referrals

Malpractice lawyer
Lurking predatorily
Awaits imprudence

ENTRIES:
A referral for
Screening sigmoidoscopy
An "innuendo"

Miles F. Adler, MD, Oakland, CA

Enter the dragon
Imperious, demanding
Difficult patient

Hugh H. Wang, MD, Pleasant Hill, CA

Managed-care system
Is managed very poorly
So we care little

Allan E. Jackman, MD, San Francisco, CA

Lost my hearing aid
Never heard of this haiku
I have not missed much

Richard K. Crissman, MD, Grand Rapids, MI

Taking colored pills
Morning, noon, and nighttime, too
Like eating money

Bernadine Z. Paulshock, MD, Wilmington, DE

Treat 'em and street 'em
That was the ER credo
Now it's don't come in

Daniel J. Colombi, MD, Haddonfield, NJ

ENT prankster
Checks right ear—sees light through left
Who has the real hole?

Joseph F. J. Curi, MD, Torrington, CT

The psychiatrist
Carefully shrinking brain cells
Oops, your time is up

Ivan Safonoff, MD, Brooklyn, NY

I say my doc's right
HMO says he is not
Guess who has to pay?

William R. McCurry, MD, Redding CA

Family doctor
Low man on the totem pole
Very high calling

Stanley Hartness, MD, Kosciusco, MS

Unexpected joy
I cauterized some skin tags
Insurance paid up

Meyer B. Hodes, MD, Oceanside, NY

HMO honcho
Collects from the rich and poor
And keeps most himself

Floyd T. Nasuti, MD, Philadelphia, PA

Team sports physician
Prepares for mayhem unknown
Prays to be used less

Stanley Rogers, DO, Oklahoma City, OK

A newborn baby
Left unnapped so carelessly
Takes this time to pee

Robert R. Jones, MD, Nevada, MO

Genetic research
Cloning of Dolly the sheep
Dolly Parton next

R. Schlein, Richmond, VA

We identify
A famous gentleman by
Peyronie's disease

Melvin J. Breite, MD, Bayside, NY

Macrosomia
Cesarean section done
No days spent in court

Jerome M. Eder, MD, Agoura, CA

Drug company rep
Feeds appetite for new drugs
And sometimes brings lunch

Randall W. Lewis, DO, Marinette, WI

A red lollipop
You braved a painful needle
Enjoy your reward

Maureen McCrum, Briarcliff Manor, NY

SQUARE FOOTERS

ASSIGNMENT:
Create a rhyming two-line medical square dance call.

EXAMPLES:

Swing your partner, do-si-do.
Don't you love your HMO?

Skip around and cross your hands
Nudge those suprarenal glands!

Couples underneath the arch
Burn that glucose (which was starch).

ENTRIES:

Promenade and form a square
If catatonic, stay right there.

Timothy J. Kutz, Kutztown, PA

Turn her back and give a squeeze
She's aspirated black-eyed peas.

Alfred D'Angelo, DO, Ormond Beach, FL

Clap you hands and give a shout
Fiddles, drown those beepers out!

Alan L. Goldman, MD, Raleigh, NC

Do-si-do and skip to my Lou
Skip a few beats, go to CCU.

Mike Ichniowski, MD, Lutherville, MD

Bow to your partner and take a dip
A good prosthesis will fix that hip.

Leo Westmoreland, MD, Hammond, LA

Round and round and round we go
Joined at the hip with an HMO.

Neal Green, MD, Corsicana, TX

Gents go underneath the ladder
Then percuss your partner's bladder.

> Anne E. Walker, MD, Charlotte, NC

Twist your back and give a nod
Then go see your orthopod.

> Morey Filler, MD, San Francisco, CA

Swing your partner to and fro
BPHers stop 'n' go.

> William Zavod, MD, Merion, PA

Grab your partner hand in hand
Informed consent they understand.

> Brian Hertz, MD, Cleveland, OH

Allemande left and promenade
Aren't you glad your deductible's paid?

> W. E. Watkins, MD, Nampa, ID

Kick those legs up off the ground
Or we'll scan your veins by ultrasound.

> Perry D. Mostov, DO, Dublin, OH

Swing your partner out and in
Don't dislodge that old hip pin.

> Herbert Gersh, MD, Treasure Island, FL

Turn your partner round about
Lift that toe if you have gout.

> Joseph Grayzel, MD, Englewood, NJ

Swing your partner round and round
Vertigo may soon abound.

> John A. Den Boer, PA-C, Walker, MI

Toss your gal, make sure you catch her
Don't you risk a Colles fracture!

David P. Perkins, MD, St. David's, PA

Four hands across, now promenade
Will we ever get paid by Medicaid?

Dr. Robert Goldberg, Lake Worth, FL

All join hands and circle the ring
Pan HMOs with a ring-a-ding-ding.

Charles G. Eschenburg, MD, Boynton Beach, FL

TO THE LETTER

ASSIGNMENT:
Resurrect and slightly amend a Latin phrase to invent a clinical meaning.

EXAMPLES:
Rima facie: A frostbitten nose
Pro bono pubico: Motto of urological association
Amicus uriae: A friendly nephrologist
Locum teens: Adolescent psychiatric disorder

ENTRIES:
AMA Mater: The mother of all medical organizations

> Charles A. Binder, MD, Toms River, NJ

Circus aximus: Improperly done circumcision

> Russell J. Cox, MD, Gastonia, NC

Ne pus ultra: Not such a bad infection

> Daniel J. Colombi, MD, Haddonfield, NJ

Ecce HMO: Bruises from fighting paymaster

> Samir Boutros, MD, South Hill, VA

Magna cart: A gurney built for two

> Ivan M. Safonoff, MD, Brooklyn, NY

Sine roles: A doctor's HMO input

> Myron Siner, MD, Wellesley, MA

Coito ergo sum: The sex addict's motto

> Pat Barwig, MD, Wauwatosa, WI

Mea ulpa: I am vomiting

> Bernadine Z. Paulshock, MD, Wilmington, DE

Quod eat demonstrandum: From the lips to the hips
Pam Johnson, Minneapolis, MN

Alter eg: Donated oocyte
Julio Novoa, MD, Perry Hall, MD

Mods operandi: Bell-bottom scrub suits
Deborah Erickson, Hershey, PA

Erra firma: An incontestable malpractice case
Joseph F. J. Curi, MD, Torrington, CT

O Tempora! O Mors!: A migraine to die for
Meyer B. Hodes, MD, East Rockaway, NY

In uturo: A fetus that's not coming out for forty weeks
Morey Filler, MD, San Francisco, CA

E pluribus num: Anesthesia for everyone
Glenn P. Lambert, MD, Flemington, NJ

Wine qua non: Chronic alcoholism
S. D. Madduri, MD, Poplar Bluff, MO

Magnum cum laud: Hyperacusis related to champagne bottle opening
Herbert Mathewson, MD, Hyannis, MA

Nodus operandi: Lymph node dissection
Joseph Szgalsky, MD, Woodbury, NJ

Contra bonos more(s): Motto of the Women Against Viagra Association
Vincent L. Keipper, MD, Concord, NC

GOOD GRACES

ASSIGNMENT:
To establish or restore goodwill with a colleague, create a phrase applicable to the profession.

EXAMPLES:
Come to terms with the obstetrician.
Scratch the dermatologist's back.
Clear the air with the pulmonologist.
Score points with the acupuncturist.

ENTRIES:
Acquiesce to humor the ophthalmologist.

Allan Plaut, MD, Lawrence, NY

Be a little patient with the pediatrician.

John S. Fox, MD, Richland, WA

Find common ground with the electrophysiologist.

Robert G. Satterfield, MD, Hermitage, TN

Make obeisances to the gynecologist.

Charles G. Eschenburg, MD, Boynton Beach, FL

Make a clean breast of things with the mammographer.

Linda Walker, MD, Columbus, GA

Be deferential to the urologist.

Bill Zavod, MD, Merion, PA

Culture the sensitivity of the microbiologist.

Kenneth M. Urban, MD, Ostrander, OH

Stroke the neurologist.

Ivan M. Safonoff, MD, Brooklyn, NY

Don't cast the first stone at the urologist.

Leo R. Westmoreland, MD, Hammond, LA

Reconciliate with the bronchoscopist.

William Broeckel, MD, Yreka, CA

Always complement the immunologist.

Marvin Barton, MD, Edison, NJ

Rectify the situation with the sigmoidoscopist.

Donald J. Sonn, MD, Springfield, MA

Ventilate with the pulmonologist.

Paul Feldham, MD, Ventura, CA

Patch things up with the plastic surgeon.

Anthony R. Russo, MD, Chesapeake, VA

Don't be put out by the anesthesiologist.

Lyn S. Aye, MD, Pasadena, CA

Get on the neurologist's wavelength.

Eva Munchnick, Ranch Palos Verdes, CA

Never rumble with the gastroenterologist.

Bernadine Z. Paulshock, MD, Wilmington, DE

Stand corrected with the orthopedic surgeon.

Alfred R. D'Angelo, DO, Ormond Beach, FL

Go with the flow with the urologist.

H. Deeths, MD, Omaha, NE

Declare a moratorium with the pathologist.

Mona Shapiro, Stockton, NJ

Avoid ticking off the parasitologist.

Patrick W. Diesfeld, MD, Ventura, CA

Avoid blow-ups with the plastic surgeon.

William G. White, MD, Franklin Park, IL

Break the impasse with the gastroenterologist.

R. Schlein, MD, Richmond, VA

Offer an infectious laugh to the epidemiologist.

Pam Johnson, RTR(BD), CDT, Minneapolis, MN

Turn the other cheek to the proctologist

Sandra B. Randolph, MD, Memphis, TN

Leland Davis, MD, Santa Rosa, CA

Allow the plastic surgeon to save face.

Aletha Oglesby, M.D., Tulsa, OK

End the blood feud with the hematologist.

Deb Randall, MA, Denver, CO

DAY JOB/NIGHT JOB

ASSIGNMENT:

If moonlighting as a professional wrestler, what nom de guerre might a health care worker adopt? And what notorious move might he use?

EXAMPLES:

The Human Centrifuge (lab technician): Whirls victims to the point of dizziness

The Lock Neck Monster (physical therapist): Applies cervical vertebral holds

Kranioklastor (obstetrician or neurosurgeon): Squeezes heads

ENTRIES:

The Wild Man of the Pampers (pediatrician): Pins opponents to the mat with safety tabs

Alan Plaut, MD, Lawrence, NY

Oedipus Rex (psychiatrist): Reduces opponent to tears by verbally attacking his mother

Morey Filler, MD, San Francisco, CA

The Abominable Toe Man (podiatrist): Stamps all over opponent after removing his corns

Gil Herzberg, MD, Larchmont, NY

The Great Scanzoni (obstetrician): Rotates heads 180 degrees

Daniel J. Colombi, MD, Haddonfield, NJ

The Venous Fly Trap (vascular surgeon): Holds and compresses legs of opponents until circulation is impaired

Nabil Dib, MD, Phoenix, AZ

Dee and Cee (OB-GYN tag team): Force opponents out of the ring, head first, while fans yell, "Push, push!"

Jonathan Ehrlich, MD, Atlanta, GA

The Ceruminator (otolaryngologist): Waxes the opposition

Allan LaReau, MD, Portage, MI

Sphincterica (g/i or g/u): The titan of tighten . . .

Michael LeVine, MD, Wimberley, TX

Lockinthar (physiatrist): Master of knees-around-neck technique.

Charles G. Eschenburg, MD, Boynton Beach, FL

Shaft (gastroenterologist): Takes rigid sigmoidoscope into ring

John B. Bassel, Jr., MD, Springfield, TN

The Flying Enema (gastroenterologist): Impact causes opponent's colonic evacuation

Russell J. Cox, MD, Gastonia, NC

Dr. Thumpenstein (cardiologist): Administers a rhythm-altering precordial thump

John Mirabello, MD, San Antonio, TX

The Terminator (HMO reviewer): Disqualifies opponent by arcane interpretation of rules

Howard T. Chatterton, MD, Ladysmith, WI

Count Dracula (venepuncturist): Immobilizes victim's arms with huge antecubital hematomas

Ivan M. Safonoff, MD, Brooklyn, NY

Angioedema Man (allergist): One touch and welts appear on victim's body.

Lisa Shakerin, MD, Robbinsdale, MN

Pseudo-Sister (lady gastroenterologist): Specialty is the "pancreatic punch."

Alton Prihoda, MD, Baytown, TX

The Human Porcupine (acupuncturist): Really sticks it to his opponents
Richard K. Crissman, MD, Grand Rapids, MI

The Sting (acupuncturist): Beware his scorpion move.
Leo Westmoreland, MD, Hammond, LA

The Facelifter (plastic surgeon): Rearranges your features
Samuel N. Grief, MD, Chicago, IL

DIAGNOSIS CONFIRMED

ASSIGNMENT:
Affix a diagnosis to explain the demise of a well-known person or group.

EXAMPLES:
Marie-Antoinette: Precipitous anencephaly
Hamlet's father: Transtympanic toxin introduction
Lot's wife: The ultimate hypernatremia
St. Valentine's Day massacre victims: Abrupt plumbism
Pompeii victims: Pneumonoultramicroscopicsilicovolcanoconiosis

ENTRIES:
Humpty-Dumpty: Unsuccessful oöcyte transfer
Michael T. McNamara, MD, High Point, NC

Medusa's victims: Reptilia-induced lithomorphism
Timothy J. Kutz, MD, Kutztown, PA

John Henry: Iron overload
B. L. Weeks, DO, Edmond, OK

Romeo and Juliet: Bilateral fatal drug error
Mariano Villasenor, MD, Pittsburgh, PA

Socrates: Hemlockjaw
William G. White, MD, Franklin Park, IL

Mata Hari: Acute lead poisoning
Bernadine Z. Paulshock, MD, Wilmington, DE

Icarus: Hyperthermic cerumenolysis with terminal velocity impact
Ivan Safonoff, MD, Brooklyn, NY

John the Baptist: Craniocervical dissociation
Daniel J. Colombi, MD, Haddonfield, NJ

Yorick: Extreme emaciation
R. C. Whitesitt, MD, Helena, MT

Bubonic plague victims: Fleabitus

Russell J. Cox, MD, Gastonia, NC

Samson: Myasthenic alopecia

Joseph F. J. Curi, MD, Torrington, CT

Samson: Quadriplegigenic pilotomy

Anatoly Belilovsky, MD, Brooklyn, NY

Sam McGee: Mixed hypothermic/hyperthermic exposure

Richard K. Crissman, MD, Grand Rapids, MI

Great Chicago Fire victims: Bovine-induced panhyperthermia

Neal Green, MD, Corsicana, TX

George Armstrong Custer: Alopecia capitis totalis

MacKenzie Smith, MD, Mercer Island, WA

Daphne: Overwhelming arborvirus

Donald S. Levi, MD, Nashua, NH

John Brown: Terminal cervical traction

David Beck, MD, Westport, CT

Julius Caesar: Septic thoracotomy

Herbert Gersh, MD, Treasure Island, FL

Julius Caesar: Brutuscellosis

Timothy J. Kutz, MD, Kutztown, PA

Prometheus: Acute intermittent millennial raptor hepatophagia

Margaret C. Rank, MD, Indialantic, FL

Joan of Arc: Fulminant hyperpyrexia

David R. Fall, MD, Gillette, WY

Wicked Witch of the East: Houseatopsus

Alton Prihoda, MD, Baytown, TX

SKIN-DEEP

ASSIGNMENT:
Create a curative patch, the first word being a nonmedical one beginning with P.

EXAMPLES:
Pisa Patch: Corrects unhealthy posture
Pub Patch: Destroys the need to overimbibe
Pig-out patch: Creates instant anorexia when overeating threatens

ENTRIES:
Phineas Fogg Patch: Prevents motion sickness for eighty days
Richard Crissman, MD, Grand Rapids, MI

Punxsutawney Patch: Informs whether reimbursement is imminent or six weeks off
Joseph B. Szgalsky, MD, Woodbury, NJ

Pooh Patch: For ursophobia
Gerald S. Roberts, MD, Lake Success, NY

Plebeian Patch: Reverses psychotic delusions of grandeur
Michael Curi, MD, Norfolk, VA

Puny Patch: Antagonistic to anabolic steroids
Alfred R. D'Angelo, DO, Ormond Beach, FL

Parka Patch: Enables coatless winter trips for hospital rounds
Bernadine Z. Paulshock, MD, Wilmington, DE

PPO Patch: Doesn't cure anything but is covered by your formulary
J. Gopin, MD, Old Bridge, NJ

Peeper Patch: Tom's transdermal therapy
Ivan M. Safonoff, MD, Brooklyn, NY

Parrot Patch: Prevents echolalia
Kathy Waller, MD, Fort Collins, CO

Potluck Patch: Who knows what you'll get?
Don Steinbrocker, MD, Los Angeles, CA

Pell-Mell Patch: Rapid conversion of catatonia
Joseph F. J. Curi, MD, Torrington, CT

Printemps Patch: Cures spring fever
Daniel J. Colombi, MD, Haddonfield, NJ

Pangloss Patch: Prevents pessimism
Timothy J. Kutz, MD, Kutztown, PA

Parent Patch: Provides Pergonal perennially
Morey Filler, MD, San Francisco, CA

P-P-P-Patch: Prevents stuttering
Stewart Sloan, MD, Omaha, NE

Pitch Patch: Enlarges the auditory frequency range
Barry Mostov, DO, Worthington, OH

Prawn Patch: Allows nonallergic fish ingestion
Michael T. McNamara, MD, High Point, NC

Plaintive Patch: Ensures more sorrowful expression for the malpractice trial jury
Jerome M. Eder, MD, Agoura, CA

Pumpkin Patch: Cures ascites and jaundice
Leora Wartofsky, MD, Tenafly, NJ

Patch Patch: Neutralizes all other patches
Ronald A. Mezger, MD, Worthington, OH

WELCOME MAT

ASSIGNMENT:
Ease a patient's anxieties in a special room with special words.

EXAMPLES:
Injection room: We'll give you our best shot.
Cystoscopy room: Urine good company
Procto room: We're behind you all the way!

ENTRIES:
Endoscopy room: We'll leave the light on!

Sidney Hartness, MD, Kosciusko, MS

Surgical pathology department: Glad to halve you!

Robert A. Ettlinger, MD, Millersburg, PA

Dietitian's counseling room: Ciao!

Timothy J. Kutz, MD, Kutztown, PA

Enema room: A straight flush beats a full house!

Edward Thompson, MD, Middletown, MD

Pulmonary function lab: If the Big Bad Wolf could do it, so can you!

Bernadine Z. Paulshock, MD, Wilmington, DE

Cath lab: We'll inject you with a warm feeling!

Joseph B. Szgalsky, MD, Woodbury, NJ

Pediatric ophthalmology suite: ICU!

Melvin J. Breite, MD, Bayside, NY

Procto room: Your posterior will be cheerier!

Daniel J. Colombi, MD, Haddonfield, NJ

Optometric suite: We're spectacular!

> Bill Zavod, MD, Merion, PA

MRI suite: Welcome to the most attractive room in the hospital!

> Richard E. Behymer, MD, Sonora, CA

X-ray room: We'll see you through!

> Sheldon Schwartz, MD, Chicago, IL

ECT room: May the force be with you!

> Arthur E. LaMontagne, MD, Manchester, CT

Mammography unit: Everybody needs a little squeeze once in a while!

> Morey Filler, MD, San Francisco, CA

Pulmonary lab: We hope you blow your test!

> Alfred R. D'Angelo, DO, Ormond Beach, FL

Lithotripsy room: We aim to ease!

> Joseph F. J. Curi, MD, Torrington, CT

Surgical suite: Come, meet the insiders!

> Hugh H. Wang, MD, Pleasant Hill, CA

Cardiology suite: Take heart!

> R. Schlein, Richmond, VA

ESWL Van: You'll have a bang-up time!

> W. E. Watkins, MD, Nampa, ID

Treadmill stress test room: We're very upbeat here!

> David Taylor, MD, Oldsmar, FL

Hemorrhoidectomy room: Come in, relax, and leave your troubled behind!

> John Mirabello, MD, Laconia, NH

MRI room: We'll pull you through!

Richard K. Crissman, MD, Grand Rapids, MI

Organ donation room: Your heart's in the right place!

Jason Felson, MD, Monroe, NY

Similarly, Carolyn T. Hall, MD, San Angelo, TX

ENTITLEMENT

ASSIGNMENT:
Choose a main literary character and diagnose him/her in modern medical terms, relating to the title.

EXAMPLES:
The Count of Monte Cristo: Nobleman with fluctuating CBC
Little Women: A batch of pituitary-deficient sisters
The Hunchback of Notre Dame: Kyphoscoliotic football star

ENTRIES:
Omoo: Mad Cow Disease

Melvin J. Breite, MD, Bayside, NY

The Compleat Angler: A case of end-stage Peyronie's disease

Richard K. Crissman, MD, Grand Rapids, MI

A Separate Peace: Siamese twins after surgery

Kathy Waller, MD, Fort Collins, CO

The Red Badge of Courage: Proud flesh

Hans W. Adams, MD, Long Beach, MS

The Sword in the Stone: Unusual open surgery for the king's urolithiasis.

Joseph B. Szgalsky, MD, Woodbury, NJ

Fahrenheit 451: Really bad hyperthermia

Dan Chiles, MD, Placentia, CA

Atlas Shrugged: A titanic case of vertebral subluxation

Miles F. Adler, MD, Oakland, CA

Prince of Tides: A man with severe polyuria

Norbert W. Leska, MD, Pennsburg, PA

The Three Musketeers: Triplets with gun-shaped ear malformations

Daniel J. Colombi, MD, Haddonfield, NJ

The Tales of Uncle Remus: One man's colonoscopy experience
Alfred R. D'Angelo, MD, Ormond Beach, FL

A Tale of Two Cities: A French radiologist's obsession with possessing two CTs
Pam Johnson, RTR, Minneapolis, MN

The Prince and the Pauper: A royal case of Cheated Twin syndrome
Michael Curi, MD, Norfolk, VA

Oliver Twist: While asking for some more gruel, child develops volvulus on top of pre-existing scoliosis
Michael Ichniowski, MD, Lutherville, MD

The Adventures of Huckleberry Finn: A boy with a cyanotic pisciform appendage
Howard F. Heller, MD, Seattle, WA

The Firm: Lawyer on Viagra
Floyd T. Nasuti, MD, Philadelphia, PA

The Prayer of Jabez: Genuflective patellar tendonitis
Yolanda J. Dreier, MD, Holly Hill, FL

Ben Hur: A transgender adventure tale
Michael A. Levine, MD, Wimberley, TX

Of Mice and Men: Pharmaceutical research team
E. Gallenstein, MD, Cincinnati, OH

The Catcher in the Rye: Baseball player with celiac sprue, noncompliant on gluten-free diet
Anthony R. Russo, MD, Chesapeake, OH

Forever Amber: Femme fatale with chronic hepatic failure
Joseph F. J. Curi, MD, Torrington, CT
Alan L. Goldman, MD, Raleigh, NC

Snow White and the Seven Dwarfs: Female albino and seven males with insufficient growth hormone

Mariano Villasenor, MD, Pittsburgh, PA

All Quiet on the Western Front: Soldiers experience profound hearing loss

Timothy J. Kutz, MD, Kutztown, PA

SPORTS AFIELD

ASSIGNMENT:

There are many sports words and phrases that could double as medical terms. Contrive a few.

EXAMPLES:

Face-off: Plastic surgeon's greatest fear
The backstretch: Physiatrist's maneuver
Three-point shot: DPT immunization
Overhead smash: Cause of subdural hematoma
Baseline: IV tubing delivering sodium bicarbonate

ENTRIES:

Ineligible receiver: HMO patient without a referral
Eli L. Rose, MD, Tampa, FL

Roughing the passer: When a patient kicks someone trying to insert a catheter
Michael J. Ichniowski, MS, Suterville, MD

Ball one, high and inside: Cryptorchidism
E. Gallenstein, MD, Cincinnati, OH

Pitch-out: Express discharge from the ambulatory surgery center
Cathy A. Krosky, MD, Amherst, OH

"He could go all the way!": Adolescent candidate for an STD
Erik Walker, MD, Winter Springs, FL

Out in left field: Out in left field
Ivan Safonoff, MD, Brooklyn, NY

Icing the puck: Prostatic cryosurgery
Charles G. Eschenburg, MD, Boynton Beach, FL

Roughing the kicker: External fetal version for breech position
Kathy Waller, MD, Fort Collins, CO

Pop fly: Initial step in urologic exam
Steven Preston, MD, Carlisle, PA

Wedge shot: Rear view of patient wearing hospital gown
Alfred R. D'Angelo, DO, Ormond Beach, FL

Fly ball: Zipper entrapment injury
Richard A. Chiarello, MD, Arlington, TX

Tip-off: Reason for malpractice claim against urologist
Ronald Olah, MD, Pasadena, CA

Grand slam: A bargain whole-body chiropractic maneuver—one move treats all
Suzanne Mahan, MD, Pueblo, CO

Suicide squeeze: Heimlich maneuver on a gorilla
Mackenzie Smith, MD, Mercer Island, WA

Fourth and two: A multipara in labor with twins
Neal Green MD, Corsicana, TX

Victory lap: Retrieval of unruptured appendix
Anne E. Walker, MD, Charlotte, NC

Bottom of the ninth: Where the taste nerve ends
Pam Johnson, RTR, Minneapolis, MN

Top seeded: In vitro fertilization recipient with the most ova
Jonathan Ehrlich, MD, Atlanta, GA

Seventh inning stretch: Striae of pregnancy
Bernadine Z. Paulshock, MD, Wilmington, DE

In field fly rule: The practice of covering the genitals during X-ray procedures
Karl M. Baumgartner, MD, Flagstaff, AZ

HANDY AITCH

ASSIGNMENT:
Insert an *H* into a medical word or term to produce a new meaning.

EXAMPLES:
Frontal shinus: Black eye
Thic douloureaux: Morbid obesity
Uterush: Pitocin effect
Wharfarin: Longshoreman's anticoagulant

ENTRIES:
Fetal hearth: A uterus

> Tejinder J. Sandhu, MD, Sanger, CA

Turph: urologist's domain

> Arthur E. LaMontagne, Jr., MD, Manchester, CT

PMSh: Being quiet while she's asleep

> Morey Filler, MD, San Francisco, CA

Thorsion: Urological emergency among the Norse gods

> Joseph B. Szgalsky, MD, Woodbury, NJ

Scholiosis: Spinal crookedness only during lectures or studying

> Brian W. Donnelly, MD, Pittsburgh, PA

Diabetes inshipidus: Hyperglycemia from cruise-related dietary excesses

> Michael Ichniowski, MD, Lutherville, MD

Ashpirator: Victim of a volcanic eruption

> Mark Donahue, MD, Mobile, AL

Chatgut: Borborygmus

> Herbert Gersh, MD, Treasure Island, FL
> Julio Novoa, MD, Perry Hall, MD

Inchision: Cut made for mini surgery
Frank P. Reynolds, MD, Jacksonville, FL

Hexanthem: Rash caused by witch doctor
Gil Herzberg, MD, Larchmont, NY

Chomplication: Lockjaw
Ellen C. Mandell, MD, Oceanside, CA

Pshoriasis: Beachgoer's dermatitis
Robert Jennette, MD, Storrs, CT

Glomerulush: Heavy drinker's kidney lesion
Steven Preston, MD, Carlisle, PA

Haxillary: Describing a poorly performed lymphadenectomy
Ron Pennington, MD, Newport Beach, CA

Handrogen: Grip-enhancing steroid
Ivan Safonoff, MD, Brooklyn, NY

Hemphysema: Lung disease from marijuana use
Deland R. Barr, DO, Weiser, ID

Chopayment: What the HMOs are doing to us
Melvin Breite, MD, Bayside, NY

Biopshy: Too small a sample
Pam Johnson, RTR, Minneapolis, MN

Penichillin: Antibiotic for the younguns
Stan Hines, MD, Huntsville, TX

Volvulush: A drunkard with vertigo
Jim Smeltzer, MD, Deerfield, OH

Thinnitus: Advanced case of anorexia
Dan W. Chiles, MD, Fullerton, CA

Hophthalmology: Study of basal brain disorder causing a peculiar gait

Robert G. Satterfield, MD, Hermitage, TN

Ghastritis: Severe stomach inflammation

R. Schlein, MD, Richmond, VA

Obsessive chompulsive: Miniscule masticator

Leland Davis, MD, Santa Rosa, CA

Hearth failure: What you get if you build a fire without opening the damper

Jay Russell, MD, Birmingham, AL

RE-VERSAL

ASSIGNMENT:
Precede the last line of a famous poem with a rhyming medical line.

EXAMPLES:
I must leave the capitations, chart review and PPO,
For the mighty wind arises, roaring seaward, and I go.
Recall yere pre-HMO life, and I'll remember mine.
We'll tak a cup o' kindness yet for auld lang syne.
HPs Dx, Labs, Rx—that is all
Ye know on earth, and all ye need to know.

ENTRIES:
I love to scope the colon's bends!
The instrument's a fright
But ah, my foes, and oh, my friends
It gives a lovely light.
(Edna St. Vincent Millay, "First Fig")

Meyer B. Hodes, MD, East Rockaway, NY

Kevorkian said, you're out of your head—just look what happened to
me . . . that night on the marge of Lake Lebarge I cremated Sam McGee.
(Robert Service, "The Cremation of Sam McGee")

Richard K. Crissman, MD, Grand Rapids, MI

Christ, if my night call were gone with the rain,
And I in my bed again.
(Anonymous, "Western Wind")

Lana L. Jeng, MD, Arvada, CO

The labor had arrested in her pelvis deep, but thanks to Caesar,
There'll be time enough to sleep.
(A. E. Housman, "Reveille")

Daniel J. Colombi, MD, Haddonfield, NJ

Denied, a claim, no pay
One word, no more, to say.
(Ralph Waldo Emerson, "Meropps")

Joseph F. J. Curi, MD, Torrington, CT

I gave up OB because of lawyers turning liars
And binding with briars my joys and desires.
(William Blake, "The Garden of Love")

Tejinder S. Sandhu, MD, Sanger, CA

The ultrasonographer bringeth light
Of things invisible to mortal sight.
(John Milton, "Light")

Russell J. Cox, MD, Gastonia, NC

Two arteries diverged at a bifurcation and I
Cathed the one less traveled by,
And that has made all the difference.
(Robert Frost, "The Road Not Taken")

Michael Ichniowski, MD, Lutherville, MD

And down with those third parties who've torn us all apart,
Who pay no praise or wages nor heed my craft or art.
(Dylan Thomas, "In My Craft or Sullen Art")

Melvin J. Breite, MD, Bayside, NY

The HMO will close its doors, we'll glad provide the lock,
When the frost is on the punkin and the fodder's in the stock.
(James Whitcomb Riley, "When the Frost is on the Punkin")

Ronald J. Pennington, MD, Newport Beach, CA

Cheers! You are dilated to eight!
Learn to labor and to wait.
(Henry Wadsworth Longfellow, "A Psalm of Life")

R. C. Whitesitt, MD, Helena, MT

My HMO has paid the bills, curing me of myriad ills,
And then my heart with pleasure fills, and dances with the daffodils.
(William Wordsworth, "I Wandered Lonely as a Cloud")

Sidney Gold, MD, Woodland Hills, CA

ON THE DECLINE

ASSIGNMENT:
Create a word or phrase specific to the practice of a colleague with jaded talents.

EXAMPLES:
Surgeon: Inoperative
Anesthesiologist: Blocked out
Nephrologist: Out of the loop.

ENTRIES:
Endoscopist: All in

Tejinder Í. Sandhu, MD, Sanger, CA

Otologist: Once waxing, now waning

Steve Burnstein, DO, Cherry Hill, NJ

Surgeon: Down for the count

Kathy Waller, MD, Fort Collins, CO

Microbiologist: Out to Pasteur

Bill Zavod, MD, Merion, PA

Bariatrician: Not pulling his weight

Bob Weeks, MD, Edmond, OK

Nephrologist: Not concentrating

Daniel J. Colombi, MD, Haddonfield, NJ

Pulmonologist: Uninspired

Michael Ichniowski, MD, Lutherville, MD

Hematologist: Spread too thin

Chris Feudtner, MD, Seattle, WA

Scrub nurse: Washed up

James P. McCann, MD, Wabash, IN

Endocrinologist: Rickety

Ronald Olah, MD, Pasadena, CA

Fertility specialist: Unproductive

Anthony R. Russo, MD, Chesapeake, VA

Pain manager: Gone to pot

Steven Preston, MD, Carlisle, PA

Neurophysiologist: Lost his potential

Anatoly Belilovsky, MD, Brooklyn, NY

Gastroenterologist: End o' scope

Jay Sivitz, MD, Jenkintown, PA

Pediatrician: Turned to the bottle

Silvia B. Vasquez, MD, Columbus, OH

Hand surgeon: Lost his grip

Steven L. Vest, MD, Norton, VA

Toxicologist: Can't get the lead out

Alfred D'Angelo, MD, Ormond Beach, FL

Cardiologist: Lost his zap

Vincent L. Kneipper, MD, Concord, NC

Chiropractor: Adjustment disorder

Gerald S. Witherell, MD, Walker, MI

Psychiatrist: Out to lunch

Bernadine Z. Paulshock, MD, Wilmington, DE

Bariatrician: Off his feed

Patricia A. Barwig, MD, Brookfield, WI

Orthopedist: Inarticulate

Alan L. Goldman, MD, Raleigh, NC

Ophthalmologist: Stye-mied

Herbert Gersh, MD, Treasure Island, FL

OB-GYN: Over the pill

Joe E. McLemore, MD, Houston, TX

Surgeon: Can't cut the mustard

Richard K. Crissman, MD, Grand Rapids, MI

Occupational health physician: Not working out

Pam Johnson, RTR, Minneapolis, MN

Dermatologist: Flaky

R. Schlein, MD, Richmond, VA

Internist: A little of all of the above

Ivan M. Safonoff, MD, Brooklyn, NY

AITCHOPENIA

ASSIGNMENT:
Drop an *H* from a medical term and provide a definition for the new word.

EXAMPLES:
Dyspagia: Reader's block
Spygmomanometer: Espionage device
Acking cough: Antiaircraft artilleryman's symptom

ENTRIES:
Weal: Beneficial urticaria

Paul B. Ross, MD, Great Neck, NY

Penylketonuria: Y-chromosome-linked metabolic disorder

Tejinder S. Sandhu, MD, Sanger, CA

Ospital: Birthing clinic

Dave Taube, Eugene, OR

Oman's sign: Patient's groan to let you know it really hurts

Kathy Waller, MD, Fort Collins, CO

Schizoprenia: Indecision at the makeup mirror

Russell J. Cox, MD, Gastonia, NC

Uretra!: Urologist's exclamation upon finding something

Hugh H. Wang, MD, Pleasant Hill, CA

Pallus: Pudendal vitiligo

Anthony R. Russo, MD, Chesapeake, VA

Dermograpia: Wine-induced erythema

Douglas Ackerman, MD, Clackamas, OR

Atropic urethritis: Dysuria in the rain forest

Ronald Olah, MD, Pasadena, CA

Ashimoto's syndrome: Consequences of a Japanese volcano
Stanley Mendelowitz, MD, Tarrytown, NY

Parmacist: Cheesemaker's knee problem
Alfred R. D'Angelo, DO, Ormond Beach, FL

Potophobia: Beer belly anxiety
Michael Curi, MD, Norfolk, VA

Litotripsy: Falling over books
Bill Zavod, MD, Merion, PA

Werdnig-Offman's disease: Killer instinct
Joel T. Appleton, MD, Abilene, TX

Neutropils: Pharmaceutical sterilization
Charles G. Eschenburg, MD, Boynton Beach, FL

Penotype: Division of male anatomic classification
Meyer B. Hodes, MD, East Rockaway, NY

AA: American Heart Association on Friday night
Mitchell A. Kopnick, MD, Janesville, WI

Andicap: Besotted bloke
Glenn P. Lambert, MD, Flemington, NJ

Glucopage: A sweet note to a loved one
Richard A. Mahrer, MD, San Jose, CA

Colangitis: Soft drink-induced vascular inflammation
Lisa Shakerin, MD, Robbinsdale, MN

MO: HMO without the health
David A. Kline, MD, Los Angeles, CA

Dyspagia: Improper use of a bookmark
Dr. Mike Holland, Texarkana, TX

Plebitis: Uprising of lower classes

Silvia B. Vasquez, MD, Columbus, OH

Metyldopa: Hard-rock groupie

Joseph F. J. Curi, MD, Torrington, CT

Epatomegaly: Progressive enlargement of pollution-controlling government agencies

Kirk R. Hassenmueller, MD, Rockingham, NC

Similarly, Hien Nguyen, MD, Fairfax, VA

Tree day Measles: Arbor Day disease

Joseph Szgalsky, MD, Woodbury, NJ

Lympocoele: An aquatic mammal with an awkward gait

George Klafter, MD, Cliffside Park, NJ

QUESTIONING QUESTIONS

ASSIGNMENT:
Provide a question so foolish that it does not require an answer.

EXAMPLES:
Nurse to doctor: "Do you want a drainage bag attached to the patient's catheter?"

Colleague to surgeon in OR lounge: "Did you finish the surgery you were doing?"

Doctor to patient leaning over basin: "Feeling sick?"

ENTRIES:
Physician to adult Siamese twins: "Do you expect me to remember everybody?"

William V. Adler, MD, Downey, CA

ER doctor to patient: "Are those Kussmaul respirations, or are you just glad to see me?"

Anatoly Belilovsky, MD, Brooklyn, NY

Unit clerk to physician running code: "You just got paged overhead. Do you want me to take a message?"

Joseph B. Szgalsky, MD, Woodbury, NJ

HMO reviewer to ER physician: "What symptoms warranted a repeat defibrillation?"

Robert Ettlinger, MD, Halifax, PA

Patient to doctor, regarding positive pregnancy test: "How did that happen?"

Aletha Oglesby, MD, Tulsa, OK

Similarly, Elizabeth A. Panzner, MD, East Hanover, NJ

Urologist to patient, after draining 1,200 cc. of retained urine: "Feel better?"

Richard K. Crissman, MD, Grand Rapids, MI

Patient to billing clerk: "Do you take cash?"

Alfred R. D'Angelo, DO, Ormond Beach, FL

Doctor to patient who just upended desk: "Can we say the Viagra is working?"

J. Marc Rosen, MD, Waianae, HI

Doctor to patient with acute red purulent inflammation: "Does it hurt when I press on it?"

Steven M. Hacker, MD, Delray Beach, FL

Secretary to doctor: "The claims are all ready to go out. Shall we send them?"

Paul B. Ross, Great Neck, NY

Doctor to nauseated patient: "How is your appetite?"

Frank J. Malta, MD, Jensen Beach, FL

Worried mother on 3:30 AM phone call to pediatrician: "Did I wake you?"

Stephen H. Mintz, MD, Syracuse, NY

Nurse to doctor after a deposition: "Did you enjoy your meeting?"

Joel T. Appleton, MD, Abilene, TX

Paramedic to patient in full arrest: "Are you OK?"

Jerome M. Eder, MD, West Hills, CA

Office clerk to doctor: "Shall I resubmit this stack of denied claims?"

Robert R. Jones, MD, Nevada, MO

Managed-care nurse to doctor: "Why does this comatose person have to be in the hospital?"

Melvin J. Breite, MD, Bayside, NY

Receptionist to man with arm in sling: "Are you here to see the doctor?"

Floyd T. Nasuti, MD, Philadelphia, PA

Patient to physician in white coat with Dermatology embroidered on it: "Are you a real doctor?"

Manfred S. Rothstein, MD, Fayetteville, NC

Nurse to unshaven, sleepy, and in scrubs resident at 4:30 AM: "Are you on call?"

Gandhi Drak, MD, Pawtucket, RI

Mother to urine-splattered pediatrician: "Can I close his diaper now, Doctor?"

Allan Plaut, MD, Lawrence, NY

AUTHOR AND OPUS

ASSIGNMENT:
Alter a renowned author's name; then create a medical book title that relates to the new name.

EXAMPLES:
Arthur Clonan Doyle: *The Coming Genetic Deluge*
Irwin Pshaw: *The Skeptic's Contrary View of Medical Literature*
Ernest Haemingway: *Dynamics of Circulation*
Louisa May Alcutt: *The Most General of General Surgery*

ENTRIES:
Sir Francid Bacon: *A Treatise on the Ptomaine*

Ivan M. Safonoff, MD, Brooklyn, NY

Emily Bronchi: *Cystic Fibrosis—A Portrait of Withering Alveoli*

Charisse Gencyuz, MD, Milan, MI

Ogden Gnash: *Living with Bruxism*

Vincent L. Keipper, MD, Concord, NC

Edgar Rice Burrholes: *Neurosurgery in a Jungle Setting*

Alan L. Goldman, MD, Raleigh, NC

Payn Rand: *Atlas Dislocated*

Steven Preston, MD, Carlisle, PA

Bram Stroker: *Effects of Blood Loss on the Cerebral Cortex*

Gene Westveer, MD, Zeeland, MI

Merck Twain: *A Manual of Medicine*

Edward A. Sciano, Jr., MD, Elmwood Park, NJ

Guy de Mo'puissant: *How to Succeed with Anabolic Steroids*

Anatoly Belilovsky, MD, Brooklyn, NY

Dr. Sues: *Thoughts on Malpractice Reversal*
> David O. Taber, MD, El Paso, TX

Danielle Steal: *The Devious Subclavians*
> Meyer B. Hodes, MD, East Rockaway, NY

Salmonella Rushdie: *A Good Picnic Wasted—The Egg Salad Chronicles*
> Richard C. Walters, MD, Webster Groves, MO

Dashiell Hamate: *A Bird in the Hand—The Story of Gamekeeper's Thumb*
> Michael Ichniowski, MD, Lutherville, MD

V. D. Salinger: *I Caught It in the Rye*
> Joseph B. Szgalsky, MD, Woodbury, NJ

Carl Sandbag: *Diagnosis of Munchausen's Syndrome*
> Joseph Grayzel, MD, Englewood, NJ

Hydrophilip Roth: *Portnoy's Dehydration*
> Steve Lieberman, MD, Clackamas, OR

Zone Grey: *A Primer of Ill-Defined Clinical Entities*
> Tejinder S. Sandhu, MD, Sanger, CA

E. L. Doctoro: *Mexican Medical Directory*
> Daniel J. Colombi, MD, Haddonfield, NJ

Voltear: *The Best New Hearing Aids*
> Randy Peck, MD, Bayside, NY

James Fenimore Scooper: *Wilderness Obstetrics*
> Joseph F. J. Curi, MD, Torrington, CT

Eugene O'Kneel: *Prepatellar Bursitis*
> Donald E. Tyler, MD, Ontario, OR

Mao Tse-Dung: *The Red Book of Scatology*
Michael Curi, MD, Norfolk, VA

Arthur Colon Doyle: *Alimentary, My Dear Watson*
Herbert Gersh, MD, Treasure Island, FL

Dr. Sauss: *Treatise on Alcoholism*
Kathy Waller, MD, Fort Collins, CO

Sir Arthur Conan Coyle: *Beyond the Pill: Newer Contraceptives*
Michael A. Levine, MD, Wimberley, TX

James Baldone: *Current Treatment of Alopecia*
Merrill Horne, MD, Midland, TX

Sallow Bellow: *Pulmonary Function in Anemics*
Gary M. Gorlick, MD, Los Angeles, CA

Langston Hues: *Tons of Dermatology Tips for Various Dermatoses*
Terri Richardson, MD, Aurora, CO

TAXES REVISITED

ASSIGNMENT:

Contrive a straight-faced medical justification of an outrageous claim to a tax auditor.

EXAMPLES:

Upscale restaurant visits: "I study the effects of gourmet fare on digestion."

Trips to Rome and Versailles: "Fountain flow rates are of vital interest to the urologist."

Years of front-row concert tickets: "I'm researching changes in the audible frequency range."

Dude ranch vacation: "I must enhance my knowledge of horseback-related prostatitis."

ENTRIES:

Stradivarius violin: "The supplier was back-ordered on tuning forks, so I had to improvise."

Steven Preston, MD, Carlisle, PA

Junkets to Las Vegas: "I'm studying carpal tunnel syndrome induced by repetitive dice-throwing."

Dave Taube, Eugene, OR

New yacht: "I need access to the hospital in case of a flood."

James R. Hoppe, MD, Piscataway, NJ

Round-the-world ocean voyage: "I'm studying the direction of vertigo above and below the equator."

Richard K. Crissman, MD, Grand Rapids, MI

World cruise: "I am studying the effects of eight meals a day on blood lipids."

Herbert Gersh, MD, Treasure Island, FL

Jewelry for wife: "I am researching heavy metal toxicity and its effects on female hormones."

S. D. Madduri, MD, Poplar Bluff, MO

A sixteen-foot $80,000 SUV: "I need to carry my Good Samaritan gear so I can help highway accident victims."

Morey Filler, MD, San Francisco, CA

Claiming all patients as dependents: "One look at the volume of office visits corroborates their dependence on me."

Michael Ichniowski, MD, Lutherville, MD

Family vacation to Disney World: "I'm a pediatric psychiatrist and I wanted to see what happy kids were like."

Melvin J. Breite, MD, Bayside, NY

Ski vacation in Aspen, Colorado: "I am writing a paper on how high-altitude pulmonary edema affects young people."

Seetha Lath, MD, Arcadia, CA

A baby grand piano: "As a surgeon, I need to keep hands and fingers limber."

R. Schlein, MD, Richmond, VA

Attending heavy metal concerts: "I am observing the seminal phase of tinnitus."

J. R. Mehta, MD, Los Angeles, CA

Multiple trips to Mexico: "I wish to show which beach resorts have the most cases of Montezuma's revenge."

Julio C. Novoa, MD, Perry Hall, MD

Two weeks at a Napa Valley inn: "I'm researching cogeners in California wines."

Ivan M. Safonoff, MD, Brooklyn, NY
Similarly, Howard S. Goldberg, MD, Southfield, MI

Beer tab: "This is a long-term study of the effects of ethanol in preventing Alzheimer's disease."

Stan Hines, MD, Huntsville, TX

Climbing the tower in Pisa: "Studying Peyronie's disease."

Timothy J. Kutz, MD, Kutztown, PA

Trip to Lourdes: "To compare the healing rate in this shrine against that of American TV evangelists."

Joel T. Appleton, MD, Abilene, TX

A relaxed pampering at the Fat Farm: "Research proving that one can eat nothing and exercise hard for a week and still gain weight as my patients swear is possible

Hugh H. Wang, MD, Pleasant Hill, CA

Seaside Resorts: "I have this friend, a pharmacist, who produces tanning lotions . . ."

Meyer Hodes, MD, E. Rockaway, NY

DRAMATIS PERSONAE

ASSIGNMENT:
From a medical word, create a lead actor in a play and describe his/her part in the drama.

EXAMPLES:
Cribriform: A lead actor who thinks he is holeyer-than-thou
Thrombus: A character who obstructs the flow of the plot
Extensor Digiti Quinti: A walk-on in a tea party scene

ENTRIES:
Calculus: A stony-faced old mathematician
Alan Goldman, MD, Raleigh, NC

Borborygmi: A small-statured actor with a dull role
Ken Urban, MD, Ostrander, OH

Pap Smear: A patriarchal political spin doctor
Michael L. Illingworth, MD, Clovis, CA

Tinea Cruris (a.k.a. Jacques Ytch): Notorious underworld nuisance
Melvin J. Breite, MD, Bayside, NY

Megaloblast: Character with a booming voice
Tejinder J. Sandhu, MD, Sanger, CA

Spermatozoon: Crowd scene extra
Daniel J. Colombi, MD, Haddonfield, NJ

Duodenum: A dynamic twosome, commonly seen wearing Levi's
Douglas Ackerman, MD, Clackamas, OH

Cremaster: An actor who muscles in and holds up the show
Morey Filler, MD, San Francisco, CA

Axilla: Odoriferous, hatchet-wielding, Tokyo-menacing giant reptile
Michael Ichniowski, MD, Lutherville, MD

Cystocoele: One who is half nun, half sea mammal
> Anthony R. Russo, MD, Chesapeake, VA

Anencephalic: Plays the Headless Horseman in a Slavic version of the *Legend of Sleepy Hollow.*
> Michael Le Vine, MD, Wimberley, TX

Tensor Veli Palatine: A high-ranged Italian tenor
> Robert G. Sullivan, MD, Boulder City, NV

Meatus: A Roman butcher who appears in the opening scene
> Deborah Abell, MD, Northampton, MA

Xenograft: A character plagued by fear of rejection
> Steven Preston, MD, Carlisle, PA

Speculum: Infiltrator who can weasel into any opening
> Joseph B. Szgalsky, MD, Woodbury, NJ

Elbow: A Hispanic suitor
> Barbara A. Matakevich, DO, Carmel, IN

Canaliculus: A rather affectionate dog
> Anatoly Belilovsky, MD, Brooklyn, NY

Priapism: An upstanding member of society
> Myron Siner, MD, Wellesley, MA
> Similarly, Richard K Crissman, MD, Grand Rapids, MI

Deltoid: One who impersonates a Mississippi native
> Michael G. Marre, MD, Rockford, IL

Metatarsus: A character who likes the footlights
> Robert Jennette, MD, Storrs, CT

WORTHY OF THE TITLE

ASSIGNMENT:
With a medical twist, alter a film title; then add a short plot synopsis.

EXAMPLES:
A Day at the Braces: Drama in the rehab ward
Scar Wars: Plastic surgeons battle over turf.
Diaboleak: Sinister force induces incontinence outbreak.

ENTRIES:
Gone with the Wound: Implantation surgeon falls into the abdominal cavity.

Joseph Grayzel, MD, Englewood

The Sound of Mucus: Ominous noise pervading ENT office

Floyd T. Nasuti, MD, Philadelphia, PA

Captain Corpulerri's Mandolin: Therapeutic strings in the bariatric clinic

John Lattin, MD, Fresno, CA

The Buns of Navarone: A liposuctionist's dream

Leonard W. Rozin, MD, Oklahoma City, OK

Don with the Wind: A flatulent Corleone turns O'Hara scarlet.

Melvin J. Breite, MD, Bayside, NY

Fetal Attraction: Obsessions in utero

Margriet Bunger, MD, McLean, VA

When Hairy Met Salty: Romance between an endocrinologically challenged couple

Frank P. Reynolds, MD, Jacksonville, FL
Robert E. Resnick, MD, Oceanside, NY

The Wizard of Schnoz: Heroic feats by plastic surgeon

Richard D. Shafron, MD, Hollywood, FL
Similarly, Ross T. Krueger, MD, Jacksonville, FL

One Flu Over the Cuckoo's Nest: Influenza epidemic compounds problems in a psychiatric ward.

Douglas Ackerman, MD, Clackamas, OR

Rash-o-man: What is the truth behind this noble couple's spots?

Jon Sudman, MD, Tucker, GA

War of the Noses: Turf war between plastic surgeons

Anthony R. Russo, MD, Chesapeake, VA

Cold Hand Luke: Raynaud's drove him to evil.

David L. Taylor, MD, Oldsmar, FL

Why a TURP?: Urologists' internecine strife over methodology

Dave Taube, MD, Eugene, OR

Diarrhea of Banned Franks: E. coli outbreak at the staff picnic

Richard K. Crissman, MD, Grand Rapids, MI

Scrutiny on the Bounty: Rich doc endures painful IRS audit.

O. Scott Lauter, MD, Lancaster, PA

The 139 Steps: Doctor applies for Medicare reimbursement

Steven Preston, MD, Carlisle, PA

Raging Bill: The gritty reality of the rising cost of health care is dramatized.

Ronald Olah, MD, Pasadena, CA

Somebody Up There Really Likes Me: Colonoscopist discovers long-stemmed roses during an exam

Daniel J. Colombi, MD, Haddonfield, NJ

Vitiligo: Alfred Hitchcock's classic story of a man who must confront his fear of hypopigmentation

Brian J. Donnelly, MD, Pittsburgh, PA

Saving Ryan's Privates

Submitted by a multitude of contributors

NEW JOB MARKET

ASSIGNMENT:
Alter a job title to create a fictional medical occupation.

EXAMPLES:
Hystorian: Gynecological archivist
Stuporvisor: Head of anesthesiology department
Gnaturalist: Tropical medicine specialist

ENTRIES:
Cornithologist: A very specialized podiatrist
Tejinder S. Sandhu, MD, Sanger, CA

Orchiologist: Infertility specialist for the older male
Alan L. Goldman, MD, Raleigh, NC

Sexophonist: On-call sex therapist
Dan W. Chiles, MD, Fullerton, CA

First braceman: Chief prosthetic technician
Bernadine Z. Paulshock, MD, Wilmington, DE

Stealworker: HMO executive
Allan LaReau, MD, Kalamazoo, MI

Buss Driver: Lip collagen injector
Morey Filler, MD, San Francisco, CA

Sirgeon: Specialist who has been knighted
Daniel J. Colombi, MD, Haddonfield, NJ

Private infestigator: STD epidemiologist
Joseph B. Szgalsky, MD, Woodbury, NJ

Vainwright: Plastic surgeon
Anatoly Belilovsky, MD, Brooklyn, NY

Cheap executive officer: Ultra-frugal hospital CEO

Alfred R. D'Angelo, DO, Ormond Beach, FL

Spinternist: White House medical spokesman

David R. Schmidt, MD, Lafayette, IN

Pleadiatrician: Child malpractice lawyer

Ed Elmensdorf, MD, Loma Linda, CA

Sproctologist: Gut-turning diagnostician

Jonathan Singer, MD, Dayton, OH

Shockbroker: Electroconvulsive therapy technician

Charles G. Eschenburg, MD, Boynton Beach, FL

Playright: Child psychiatrist

Andreas D. Sideridis, MD, Flushing, NY

Taxicologist: Specialist in heavy traffic CO fumes

Lazaro E. Javier, MD, Sandusky, MI

Cadministrator: hospital director

Carole Macaulay, MD, La Habra Heights, CA

Barriotrician: A doctor practicing in an underserved area

Robert A. Gerber, MD, Sherman Oaks, CA

Fiscal therapist: Hospital CPA

Jerry Billmeier, MD, Memphis, TN

Paleoncologist: Student of ancient tumors

Meyer Hodes, MD, East Rockaway, NY

Prostatute: Medico-legal urologist

Ronald Olah, MD, Pasadena, CA

Ticnician: Facial nerve specialist

William P. Klein, MD, Orangeburg, NY

Lumbarjack: Orthopedic spinal specialist
Mackenzie Smith, MD, Mercer Island, WA

Peeanist: Musical urologist
S. D. Madduri, MD, Poplar Bluff, MO
Rudi Kirschner, MD, Phoenix, AZ

Hinternist: Rural-based diagnostician
Jeffery T. Wu, MD, Newton, MA

Vendocrinologist: Prepaid glandular disorder specialist
Stan Morrison, MD, Lodi, CA

SPLITSVILLE

ASSIGNMENT:
Alter a medical word or expression by adding a space to form new words. Then define the words.

EXAMPLES:
A trial flutter: Let's test those baby blues!
Bet a blocker: Okay, and I'll wager a running back!
Oo Genesis!: Reaction of seminarians given a surprise quiz on the Old Testament

ENTRIES:
Broncho spasm: The most exciting part of the rodeo
Robert Ettlinger, MD, Halifax, PA

Syn apse: A section of the church vestibule for those coming together to repent
Richard B. Stewart, MD, Doraville, GA

Vas it is?: Vy you vant to know?
Meyer B. Hodes, MD, East Rockaway, NY

Diver ticulum: Nitrogen narcosis-induced scuba giggles
Karen Larson, MD, Littleton, CO

Thy roid: Where thou puttest ye Preparation H
Raffi Krikorian, MD, Swansea, IL

Men o pause!: . . . and contemplate the wonders of life
Pam Johnson, RTR, Minneapolis, MN

Ex udate: Attempt to rekindle a lost romance
Russell J. Cox, MD, Gastonia, NC

Cor pus callosum: A really big heart infection
Cecil Jenkins, MD, Jackson, MS

Auto graft: Pricey car driven by corrupt public official
Mariano Villaseñor, MD, Pittsburgh, PA

My ring it is: No, it's not your pager!
R. Joseph Paquette, MD, Spring Hill, FL

He art beat: Shakespeare loses
Valerie Goldfain, MD, Kankakee, IL

In continent: The land mass with the latest boutiques
Deborah Erickson, MD, Hershey, PA

Ex anthem: A song formerly sung in honor of one's country
E. Gallenstein, MD, Cincinnati, OH

Chord ee: Asynchronous musical variation for the urologist
Joseph F. J. Curi, MD, Torrington, CT

Mo no blast: Mets slugger goes homerless
Daniel J. Colombi, MD, Haddonfield, NJ

A cute mast it is: Martha Stewart describes her decorated sloop
Newton B. Miller, MD, Norfolk, VA

Pre puce: Not blue, not violet
Alfred R. D'Angelo, DO, Ormond Beach, FL

Fun gal infection: Consequences of unprotected sex
Stanley Mendelowitz, MD, Tarrytown, NY

O vary: Egg salad sandwich, hold the mayo
Morey Filler, MD, San Francisco, CA

Dis section: A part of de town where one should not walk at night
Leonard C. Eppard, MD, Lorton, VA

FACE THE MUSIC

ASSIGNMENT:
Choose a piece of music and, in a medical sense, describe what it is about.

EXAMPLES:
The Pathetique: Doctor petitioning for fair reimbursement
Danse Macabre: Theme social for forensic pathologists
Apassionata: Specialists railing against malpractice premium hike
The Archduke Trio: Group doing foot and hand surgery

ENTRIES:
Haydn's Surprise Symphony: Dr. Haydn bills HMO $2,751.24; HMO pays Dr. Haydn $2751.24.

Jonathan S. Ehrlich, MD, Atlanta, GA

Götterdämmerung: Tinnitus complaint

Joseph F. J. Curi, MD, Torrington, CT

"Deh vieni, non tardar": Plea of patients whose MD is more than an hour late

Janna Peake, MD, Arden Hills, MN

Five Lieder, Op. 40: Request for more blood in operating room 40

Lana L. Jeng, MD, Arvada, CO

"La donna e mobile": Your female patient can ambulate, so discharge her.

Meyer Hodes, MD, Rockaway, NY

Royal Fireworks Music: Laparoscopic electrosurgery gone awry

Peyman Zandieh, MD, Bethpage, NY

The Pearl Fishers Duet: Two academic physicians on rounds at the medical center

Ed Lamon, MD, Albuquerque, NM

Dance of the Apprentices: First day of internship
Lisa Shakerin, MD, Robbinsdale, MN

March to the Scaffold: Unprepared applicant about to begin oral certification exam
Daniel J. Colombi, MD, Haddonfield, NJ

Traumerei: Another corneal abrasion in the emergency room
Melvin Breite, MD, Bayside, NY

Adagio, 1st Movement: Chronic constipation
Allan LaReau, MD, Kalamazoo, MI

The Anvil Chorus: Choir at the otology convention
Richard K. Crissman, MD, Grand Rapids, MI

The Beggar's Opera: Music heard while on hold for HMO's claim-denial line
Michael Curi, MD, Norfolk, VA

La Nozze di Figaro: Italian man's rhinoplasty
Glenn P. Lambert, MD, Flemington, NJ

Purgatorio: Enema room
Tejinder J. Sandhu, MD, Sanger, CA

Echo et Narcisse: Schizophrenic recurrently hearing, "You are the best"
Shashi K. Agarwal, MD, Orange, NJ

West Side Story: The search for suitable medical office space
R. Schlein, MD, Richmond, VA

The Nutcracker Suite: Where vasectomies and/or lobotomies are performed
J. W. Budell, MD, Stone Mountain, GA

Madame Butterfly: Female ER doctor who eschews sutures and staples
Floyd T. Nasuti, MD, Philadelphia, PA

HANG-UPS

ASSIGNMENT:
Conceive of a windshield knickknack suspended from the rear-view mirror that proclaims one's specialty.

EXAMPLES:
Surgeon: Crossed swords
Forensic pathologist: Skull and crossbones
Otologist: Drum

ENTRIES:
Alternative medicinist: Eye of newt, lizard's leg, tooth of wolf
Joseph F. J. Curi, MD, Torrington, CT

Lithotripsist: Kidney-shaped stone and stick of dynamite
Tejinder S. Sandhu, MD, Sanger, CA

Pediatric ophthalmologist: One letter *I* across another
Alan L. Goldman, MD, Raleigh, NC

Hockey team dentist: False teeth with central incisors missing
Daniel J. Colombi, MD, Haddonfield, NJ

Psychiatrist: Shrunken head and hourglass
Stanley Hartness, MD, Kosciusko, MS

Allergist: Miniature nasal inhaler and a red swollen nose
Delores A. Corpuz, MD, Carrollton, TX

Pathologist: Toe tags and formalin air freshener
Amy Chai, MD, Ellicott City MD

Podiatrist: Large foot with corn kernels on toes
Parricia J. Fogle, DO, Berea, KY

Obstetrician: Catcher's mitt
Stephen L. Burnstein, DO, Cherry Hill, NJ

Cardiologist: King of Hearts playing card

Michael J. Gordon, MD, Houston, TX

Proctologist: Rear-view mirror

David L. Anders, MD, Peachtree City, GA

Internist: Caduceus formed by a stethescope wrapped around a pen

Vincent Keipper, MD, Concord, NC

Neurologist: Ticking clock

Morey Filler, MD, San Francisco, CA

Otolaryngologist: Pony (a little horse) with a frog in its mouth

Alan R. Prihoda, MD, Baytown, TX

Anesthesiologist: Pair of fuzzy *Z*s skewered by a spinal needle

L. S. Aye, MD, Auburn, CA

Spinal surgeon: Bobblehead

Irving Thorne, MD, Bloomington, MN

Plastic surgeon: Half a dozen different-shaped noses

Michael E. Trigg, MD, Wilmington, DE

Psychiatrist: A cracked pot

Richard K. Crissman, MD, Grand Rapids, MI

Psychiatrist: Bag of nuts

Floyd T. Nasuti, MD, Philadelphia, PA

ECT psychiatrist: Plastic lightning bolt

Joseph Szgalsky, MD, Woodbury, NJ

RHYME TIME

ASSIGNMENT:
Name someone in the medical field with two rhyming words that describe his/her job.

EXAMPLES:
Psychiatrist specializing in alcoholism: Drink shrink
Very laid-back bariatrician: Looser reducer
Reluctant TUR surgeon: Objectionist resectionist
Nervous obstetrician: Quiverer deliverer

ENTRIES:
Clumsy hand surgeon: Palmer harmer
> Melvin J. Breite, MD, Bayside, NY

Urologist treating Peyronie's: Bender mender
> O. Scott Lauter, MD, Lancaster, PA

Orthopedist to the clergy: Pastor caster
> Steven Preston, MD, Elizabethtown, KY

Physician-attorney: Tort sort
> Daniel J. Colombi, MD, Haddonfield, NJ

Hospital-based doctor: Insider provider
> Richard K. Crissman, MD, Grand Rapids, MI

Pharmacist: Elixir fixer
> William B. Owen, Jr., MD, Waynesville, NC

Sartorially correct laser retinologist: Dapper zapper
> Philip J. Frankenfeld, Ph.D., Washington, DC
> Similarly, Herbert Gersh, MD, Treasure Island, FL

Non-American pathologist: Foreigner coroner
> Pat Landry, MD, Seneca, SC

Treater of Parkinsonians: Tremor stemmer
William Steffan, MD, Laguna Beach, CA

British ENT doing nasal anesthesia: Coke bloke
Jon Sudman, MD, Tucker, GA

One of vanishing breed of male OB-GYNs: Mr. Hyster
Morey Filler, MD, San Francisco, CA

Electrocardiographer: Pacer tracer
Shashi K. Agarwal, MD, Orange, NJ

Dermabrading plastic surgeon: Peeler healer
Pepi Granat, MD, South Miami, FL

Fracture-stabilizing orthopedist: Bracer placer
Neal Green, MD, Corsicana, TX

Insomnia primary physician: Sleepy GP
Jerry Billmeier, MD, Memphis, TN

Speech pathologist on house calls: Walkie-talkie
Mary Ann McTiernan, Wayne, NJ
Patricia Fogle, DO, Berea, KY

Unenlightened dermatologist: Simpler pimpler
Perry D. Mostov, DO, Worthington, OH

Obese code team member: Plumper thumper
Joseph B. Szgalsky, MD, Woodbury, NJ

Cryogenic geriatrician: Geezer freezer
Bill Zavod, MD, Merion, PA

Eye surgeon: Visionary incisionary
Ronald Olah, MD, Pasadena, CA

Casino employees' health doctor: Dealer healer
R. C. Rau, MD, no address

Urologist specializing in incontinence: Leak freak

Andreas D. Sideridis, MD, Flushing, NY

Geriatric pulmonologist: Geezer wheezer appeaser

Barton Perry, MD, Centre, AL

Well-mannered surgeon: Proper chopper

Gil Herzberg, MD, Larchmont, NY

Adept phlebotomist: Quicker slicker pricker

Jack Cole, MD, Bethlehem, PA

QUADRIPEDICS

ASSIGNMENT:
Link a medical person's pet's name with the owner's type of work.

EXAMPLES:
HMO Executive: Buck
Ophthalmologist: Blinky
Hand surgeon: Duke

ENTRIES:
Gynecologist: Menopaws

> Clifford A. Gordon, MD, Wayne, NJ

Cardiologist: QRST (pronounced *Christie*)

> Shashi K. Agarwal, MD, Orange, NJ

Proctologist: Assta

> Arthur LaMontagne, Jr., MD, Manchester, CT

Vascular surgeon: Bluetoe

> Steve Lieberman, MD, Clackamas, OR

HMO gatekeeper: Pushinka

> Daniel Schual-Berke, MD, Seattle, WA

Medical billing clerk: FeeFee

> Carey S. Goltzman, MD, Chappaqua, NY

Radiologist's cat: Scan

> Ashlesha Tamboli, MD, Minneapolis, MN

Orthopedic surgeon: Rodknee

> Douglas Wadeson, MD, Satellite Beach, FL

Urologist: Einstein

> Meyer B. Hodes, MD, East Rockaway, NY

Electrophysiologist: Voltaire

Nabil Dib, MD, Phoenix, AZ

Medical coder: K-9

Andreas D. Sideridis, MD, Flushing, NY

Chief of staff: King

Frank P. Reynolds, MD, Jacksonville, FL

Venerealogist: Louise

Alan L. Goldman, MD, Raleigh, NC

Substance abuse specialist: Tippler

R. Schlein, MD, Richmond, VA

Neurologist: Twitch

Jesse Hackell, MD, Pomona, NY

Proctologist: Uranus

Ruben Victores, MD, Beaumont, TX

Urologist: E-Rex

James R. Fishman, MD, Phoenix, AZ

Forensic investigator doctor of osteopathy: FIDO

Allan LaReau, MD, Kalamazoo, MI

Sexual therapist: Floppy

Alfred R. D'Angelo, MD, Ormond Beach, FL

Trauma surgeon: Wrecks

Melvin Breite, MD, Bayside, NY

Gynecologist: G-spot

Julio C. Novoa, MD, Perry Hall, MD

Neurosurgeon: Koko

John Lattin, MD, Fresno, CA

Oncologist: Kimo

> Charles G. Eschenburg, MD, Boynton Beach, FL

Podiatrist: Archie

> Herbert Gersh, MD, Treasure Island, FL

Podiatrist: Achilles

> Lisa C. Gold, MD, Crown Point, IN

Gastroenterologist: Gutsy

> S. Bharath, MD, Devil's Lake, ND

Numerous contributors rendered the following:

Cardiologist: Thumper
Gynecologist: Spot
Locum tenens doc: Rover

AUTOLOGOUS

ASSIGNMENT:
Adjust a car title and match it to its driver's line of medical work.

EXAMPLES:
Elderado: Geriatrician
Plexus: Neurologist
Incontinental: Urologist
Cutless: Laser surgeon

ENTRIES:
Cheep Wrangler: HMO executive

Alan G. Plaut, MD, Lawrence, NY

Rales Royce: Pulmonologist

David Taube, Eugene, OR

Dodge DaQuota: Hospital administrator

David C. Allen, MD, Twin Falls, ID

Carvette: Female surgeon

Richard K. Crissman, MD, Grand Rapids, MI

Acurare: Anesthesiologist

Russell J. Cox, MD, Gastonia, NC

Heclipse: Circumcisionist

Gloria R. Julius, St. Petersburg, FL

Slaab: Pathologist

Andreas D. Sideridis, MD, Flushing, NY

Yugo: Hospital PRO physician

Shashi K. Agarwal, MD, Orange, NJ

Fjord Sexcurgeon: Scandinavian HIV specialist

William Steffan, MD, Laguna Beach, CA

Gutlass: Female gastroenterologist

Stephen L. Burnstein, D.O., Cherry Hill, NJ

Chevy Capricious: Malpractice lawyer

Suzanne Mahan, MD, Pueblo, CO

Laserati: Italian ophthalmologist

Bernadine Z. Paulshock, MD, Wilmington, DE

Winnelumbago: Orthopedist

Richard Silberg, MD, Baltimore, MD

Toyota Mamry: Plastic surgeon

Michael Ichniowski, MD, Lutherville, MD

Studemaker: Infertility specialist

Kathy Waller, MD, Fort Collins, CO

Gnash: Oral surgeon

John G. Black, MD, Columbia, SC

Croup De Ville: House pediatrician

Daniel J. Colombi, MD, Haddonfield, NJ

Miatus: Urologist

Ivan Safonoff, MD, Stockton, NJ

Cadillac Catarrha: Otolaryngologist

Bora Kim, MD, Thousand Oaks, CA

Limberghini: Physical therapist

Micheal Selby, MD, Little Rock, AR

Lumbargenie: Back surgeon

Lisa Shakerin, MD, Robbinsdale, MN

Subaru Cutback: Hospital or HMO CEO

Michael Ichniowski, MD, Lutherville, MD

Scentury: Rhinoplasty specialist

Luann Woods, DO, Tulsa, OK

Vulvo: Gynecologist

David Perkins, MD, St. Davids, PA

Testosterrosa: Endocrinologist/urologist

Newton B. Miller, MD, Norfolk, VA

Camarrow: Oncologist

Pam Johnson, RTR, Minneapolis, MN

Crown Dictoria: Urology department head

Irving Thorne, MD, Minneapolis, MN

Priaprizm: Urologist

Eric Strauss, MD, Palo Alto, CA

MYTHELLANEOUS

ASSIGNMENT:
Attribute a medical connection to a mythical character's name.

EXAMPLES:
Sir Lancelot: The master of the I & D
Venus: Phlebotomist
Phoebus: Transportation for the underpaid to protest at managed care GHQ
Loki: Understated physician

ENTRIES:
Phoenix: Insurance claim adjuster
> Dave Taube, Eugene, OR

Thor: Failed New York cryotherapist
> Morey Filler, MD, San Francisco, CA

Castor and Pollux: Purgative rule of thumb
> G. J. Billmeier, MD, Memphis, TN

Icarus: Collective reaction to draining pilonidal sinus
> James Ulery, MD, Monroe, MI

Hebe: Patient whose nervous condition is manifest by the presence of her brother, Jebe
> J. R. Mehta, MD, Los Angeles, CA

Minerva: A small neurologist
> Steven Preston, MD, Elizabethtown, KY

Io: Medical student
> Lyn S. Aye, MD, Auburn, CA
> Similarly, Stephen L. Kaufman, MD, San Francisco, CA

Euterpe: Urologist at work

Douglas Ackerman, MD, Clackamas, OR

Roc: Lithotripsy technician

Amy Porter, MD, La Canada, CA

Pales: HMO credo

Joseph F. J. Curi, MD, Torrington, CT

Porus: The underpaid physicians in managed care

Daniel J. Colombi, MD, Haddonfield, NJ

Erato: Physician reviewer for HMOs

Charles Webb, MD, Traverse City, MI

Zeus: Publisher of paper on green eggs and ham

Mark Abel, MD, Brick, NJ

Hippolyta: Liposuction master

Lisa Shakerin, MD, Robbinsdale, MI

Boreas: A dull medical professor

Vincent L. Keipper, MD, Concord, NC

Pan: General practitioner

R. Schlein, MD, Richmond, VA

Minos: Rhinoplasty surgeon

Mary McTiernan, Wayne, NJ

Euripides: Causer of wound dehiscence

David E. Schoenfeld, MD, Carrollton, GA

Bacchus: Expert MDs for the defense

V. A. Short, MD, Ellisville, MD
Suzanne E. Mahan, MD, Pueblo, CO

Sir Kay (foster brother of King Arthur): Potassium replacement specialist

Shashi K. Agarwal, MD, Orange, NJ

Urania: Nuclear medicine specialist

Michael Curi, MD, Norfolk, VA

Demosthenes: Exhibitor of prepared joint prosthesis

Mike Holland, MD, Texarkana, TX

THE CLINICAL TEAM

ASSIGNMENT:
Match the name of a sports team to an appropriate medical participant.

EXAMPLES:
Big Red: Allergists
Pacers: Cardiologists
Crimson Tide: Obstetricians/gynecologists
Islanders: Diabetologists

ENTRIES:
Fighting Sioux: Clinic risk-management committee
Deanne Johnson, MD, Park Rapids, MN

Macon Whoopee: Sex therapists
Seth Hirschfield, MD, Cleveland, OH

Ramblin' Wrecks: Gerontologists
Michael Szymanski, MD, Dexter, MI

Hammerheads: Neurosurgeons
Charles G. Eschenburg, MD, Boynton Beach, FL

Privateers: Urologists
David Taube, Eugene, OR

Dodgers: HMO billing officers
Gilbert Herzberg, MD, Larchmont, NY

Celtics: Lyme disease researchers
Anthony R. Russo, MD, Chesapeake, VA

Red Raiders: Phlebotomists
Russell J. Cox, MD, Gastonia, NC

Orangemen: Vitamin A researchers
Neal Green, MD, Corsicana, TX

Golden Flashes: Geriatric gynecologists

Joseph F. J. Curi, MD, Torrington, CT

Daniel J. Colombi, MD, Haddonfield, NJ

Braves: Physicians still practicing in Pennsylvania or Florida

Alfred R. D'Angelo, DO, Ormond Beach, FL

V. A. Short, MD, Ellisville, MS

Badgers: Hospital security guards

Frank P. Reynolds, MD, Jacksonville, FL

Commodores: Colorectal surgeons

Douglas Ackerman, MD, Clackamas, OR

As: Successful premedical students

Melvin Breite, MD, Bayside, NY

Roadrunners: Ambulance attendants

Patricia Fogle, DO, Berea, KY

Sharks: MD /JD malpractice plaintiff attorneys

David Tuerk, MD, Palo Alto, CA

Blue Devils: Pulmonologists

H. Bruce Daniels, MD, Cleburne, TX

Pistons: Urologists

Mark L. Fallick, MD, Voorhees, NJ

Cornhuskers: Podiatrists

Sam Moorer, MD, Tallahassee, FL

James M. Friedman, MD, Fort Worth, TX

Devil Rays: Radiologists

Allan B. Solum, MD, Paynesville, MN

Sooners: Neonatologists:

Aletha Oglesby, MD, Tulsa, OK

Golden Gophers: Senior medical students
                    Daniel M. Hoffman, MD, Fredericksburg, VA

Lugnuts: Overworked psychiatrists
                    Richard K. Crissman, MD, Grand Rapids, MI

Wizards: PhD, MD

                    Martin W. Stallings, MD, Kings Mountain, NC

Warthogs: Dermatologists
                    Joseph Kloss, MD, Akron, OH

Pistons: HMO-affiliated physicians
                    Howard S. Goldenberg, MD, Southfield, NJ

Many contributed these two names:
    Mets: Oncologists
    Trojans: Family planning or sex therapists

NURSING RHYMES

ASSIGNMENT:
Choose a nursery rhyme and compose a medically slanted second line.

EXAMPLES:
Diddle diddle dumpling, my son John
Lasered his own chalazion
Old King Cole was a merry old soul
'Til senile dementia took its toll
To market, to market, to buy a fat pig
Beware trichinosis, a risk that is big

ENTRIES:
As I was going to St. Ives, I met a man with seven wives
All on their way to Inverness, to find a cure for PMS.

Anatoly Belilovsky, MD, Brooklyn, NY

Old MacDonald had a farm, Ee-i-ee-i-oh
He also had dyslexia, ho-i-ee-i-ee.

Julio Novoa, MD, Perry Hall, MD

Little Boy Blue, come blow your horn
Our audiometer died this morn.

Dan W. Chiles, MD, Placentia, CA

The green bug sleeps in a white lily ear
Its plasmid resistance is something we fear.

James Smith, MD, Gilbert, AZ

Jack be nimble, Jack be quick
End my aching, I'm too sick.

Joseph F. J. Curi, MD, Torrington, CT

The itsy-bitsy spider went up the waterspout
After the TURP, he came a-flying out.

Steven Preston, MD, Elizabethtown, KY

Mary, Mary, quite contrary, how does your garden grow?
The cannabis is doing well, as all my addicts know.

Richard K. Crissman, MD, Grand Rapids, MI

Ride a cock horse to Banbury Cross
You'll be admitted to Psych, of course.

Meyer B. Hodes, MD, East Rockaway, NY

As I went over Lincoln Bridge
I slipped and cracked my petrous ridge.

John Lattin, MD, Fresno, CA

Jack and Jill went up the hill to fetch a pail of water
Jack fell down and broke his crown, was burrholed by his (neurosurgeon)
daughter.

Josef Vosmek, MD, Strum, WI

I do not like thee, Dr. Fell
I paid your fee, still I'm not well.

Daniel J. Colombi, MD, Haddonfield, NJ

Georgie Porgie, puddin' and pie
Could not enjoy it—had a Roux-en-Y.

Alton R. Prihoda, MD, Baytown, TX

Kookaburra sits in the old gum tree
Alzheimer's set in, of moderate degree.

Shashi K. Agarwal, MD, Orange, NJ

Now I lay me down to sleep
Assured to wake because of PEEP.

Ivan Safonoff, MD, Stockton, NJ

Three blind mice, three blind mice
Didn't use their Xalatan—bad advice.

Bob Weeks, DO, Edmond, OK

Pease porridge hot, pease porridge cold
Watch out for E. coli when it's nine days old.

Paul Lucca, MD, Milwaukee, WI

Mary had a little lamb, its fleece was white as snow
That anthrax lay concealed within, this Mary did not know.

Ophelia J. Mall, MD, Flemington, NJ

There was a crooked man and he walked a crooked mile
They cured his scoliosis, now he wears a crooked smile.

Norman D. Lindley, MD, Alomogordo, NM

HELP IS ON THE WAY

ASSIGNMENT:
Come up with a remedy in rhyme for a suffering traveler in a foreign place.

EXAMPLES:
A brace in Thrace
Vermifuge at the Moulin Rouge
Optic rinse in Port-au-Prince
Prostatic massage at the Hermitage

ENTRIES:
A Swan-Ganz in Cannes, France

Michael Ichniowski, MD, Lutherville, MD

T&A in Saint-Tropez

Stanley S. Paras, MD, Bedford, NH

Penile prosthesis in the Peloponnessus

Richard Silberg, MD, Baltimore, MD

Epidurals in the Urals

Jay Mehta, MD, Los Angeles, CA

Lamaze in LaPaz

Peyman Zandieh, MD, Bethpage, NY

Iron lung in Kwangtung

Joseph F. J. Curi, MD, Torrington, CT

Tubal tie in old Shanghai

Bernadine Z. Paulshock, MD, Wilmington, DE

Ice and heat in Canea, Crete

Morey Filler, MD, San Francisco, CA

Yank a drain in Alsace-Lorraine
Deborah K. Walland, MD Hilton Head, SC

Fix uterine descent in the Fertile Crescent
Vincent L. Keipper, MD, Concord, NC

Transplant a kidney from Melbourne to Sydney
Robert Ettlinger, MD, Halifax, PA

CPR in Zanzibar
Steven Preston, MD, Elizabethtown, KY

Induce in Belarus
Karen Jakpor, MD, Riverside, CA

Unna boot in Beirut
Catherine Biren, MD, Modesto, CA

Diaphragm in Amsterdam
Daniel J. Colombi, MD, Haddonfield, NJ

Chicken soup in Guadalupe
Gloria R. Julius, St. Petersburg, FL

Drain the belly in New Delhi
Richard K. Crissman, MD, Grand Rapids, MI

Fen-phen in Phnom Penh
Shashi K. Agarwal, MD, Orange, NJ

Root canal at the Taj Mahal
Mariano Villasenor, MD, Pittsburgh, PA

A cortisone shot in Montserrat
Peter Stahl, MD, Columbia, SC

Cervical freeze in Belize
Vincent Napoliello, MD, Wayne, NJ

A dorsal slit in Tikrit

Douglas Ackerman, MD, Clackamas, OR

Gastric lavage at Lake LaBarge

Mackenzie Smith, MD, Mercer Island, WA

Heimlich maneuver in Vancouver

R. Schlein, MD, Richmond, VA

A vasodilator in Ulan Bator

Floyd T. Nasuti, MD, Philadelphia, PA

A tummy tuck in Innsbruck

Marilyn B. Price, RN, Gonzales, TX

SPECIALTY OF THE HOUSE

ASSIGNMENT:
Slightly alter a menu item so that it is appropriate for a diner who is a doctor.

EXAMPLES:
Vascular surgeon: Clamp chowder
Rheumatologist: Baba au rheum
Neurologist: Seizure salad
Cryotherapist: Enchilladas

ENTRIES:
In-vitro specialist: Egg McStuffin
Melvin J. Breite, MD, Bayside, NY

Cardiorespiratory physician: Heartichokes
Patricia J. Fogle, DO, Berea, KY

Podiatrist: Corn on the job
Yan Chow, MD, Pleasanton, CA

Endocrinologist: Lobster thermendorph
Dave Taube, Eugene, OR

Hospital administrator: Poorhouse steak
Andreas D. Sideridis, MD, Flushing, NY

Neurologist: Flounder Ménière
Daniel J. Colombi, MD, Haddonfield, NJ

Bariatrician: Leaner schnitzel
Joseph F. J. Curi, MD, Torrington, CT

Ophthalmologist: Eye screen sundae
Scott Siegel, MD, East Brunswick, NJ

Reproductive technologist: Him 'n' eggs

Morey Filler, MD, San Francisco, CA

Neurologist: Beef strokeanoff

Russell J. Cox, MD, Gastonia, NC

HMO physician: Po' boys

Stanley Rogers, D.O., Oklahoma City, OK

Plastic surgeon: Faked Alaska

Steven Preston, MD, Elizabethtown, KY

MD/JD doing malpractice: Sue she

Allan LaReau, MD, Kalamazoo, MI

Dietitian: Carb salad

Amy Porter, MD, La Canada, CA

Child psychiatrist: Bratwurst

Bill Zovod, MD, New York, NY

Bob Rau, MD, Columbus, OH

Medicare assignment acceptors: Potatoes au gratis

Allan B. Solum, MD, Paynesville, MN

Spinal orthopedist: Jamdalumba

Hugh H. Wang, MD, Concord, CA

Laparoscopist: Trendelenburgers

Lisa Shakerin, MD, Robbinsdale, MN

Urologist: Wienerschpritzl

Richard Silberg, MD, Baltimore, MD

Psychiatrist: Southern Freud chicken with Jung baby vegetables

Kathryn Watkins, Gastonia, NC

Infertility specialist: Eggs ovariesy

Michael Ichniowski, MD, Lutherville, MD

Reproductive endocrinologist: Donor eggs Benedict
David Orenstein, MD, Paradise Valley, AZ

Urologist: Slow peas
Brent W. Allain, MD, Franklin, LA

Orthopedist: Patella a la Valenciana
Julio C. Novoa, MD, Perry Hall, MD

Space physician: Oysters Rocketfeller
Vincent L. Keipper, MD, Concord, NC

Burn specialist: Sizzling Happy Family (Chinese Dish)
Amy Lemley, Charlottesville, VA

Ophthalmologist: Peking duct
J. R. Mehta, MD, Los Angeles, CA

Chinese endocrinologist: Peking duct
Douglas Ackerman, MD, Clackamas, OR

WHAT WAS THAT YOU SAID?

ASSIGNMENT:
Guess at a patient's interpretation of a medical term heard for the first time.

EXAMPLES:
Inguinal ring: A phone call to discuss hernia repair methods
Plaster of Paris: ER term for intoxication by french wines
Mastectomy: A nautical crisis

ENTRIES:
Aqueous humor: The old clown flower trick
Vincent I. Keipper, MD, Concord, NC

Anastomoses: Biblical reference to giving Moses a donkey
David A. Kline, MD, Los Angeles, CA

Ataxic: Unable to hail a cab
Dan Colombi, MD, Haddonfield, NJ

Roux-en-Y: A glass of red wine at the YMCA
Neal Green, MD, Corsicana, TX

Menometrorrhagia: Angry men on the subway
Heidi M. McNaney-Flint, MD, Stuart, FL

Munchausen syndrome: Compulsion to emulate termites
Dan Chiles, MD, Fullerton, CA

Penile erection: A solution to jail overcrowding
Alex Fishberg, MD, Wabash, IN

Lactose intolerant: Unable to abide the digitally impaired
Floyd T. Nasuti, MD, Philadelphia, PA

Myringotomy: What I had done when my finger grew too fat for ring removal

Michael Meyer, MD, Roanoke, VA

SOB: Family wondering how note-taking intern knew their dyspneic father so well

Cason De La Houssaye, MD, Crowley, LA

Charcot's joint: A French bistro

Alan L. Goldman, MD, Raleigh, NC

Grand mal seizure: Compulsive urge to shop at the galleria

Jay Malhotra, MD, Burr Ridge, IL

Cauterize: Made visual contact

S. D. Madduri, MD, Poplar Bluff, MO

Brachytherapy: A course given to speeders

Robert A. Edelman, MD, Garden City, NY

URI: No, you are you. I am me.

Jan Sudman, MD, Tucker, GA

VP shunt: Choice of a new running mate at the last minute

Steven Preston, MD, Elizabethtown, KY

Oocyte: Awesome scenic attraction

Penny I. Burdick, MD, Issaquah, WA

Caruncle: Relative who refuses to walk

Herbert Gersh, MD, Treasure Island, FL

Leukopenia: Hitman in *Godfather IV*

Joseph F. J. Curi, MD, Torrington, CT

His Bundle study: Evaluation of male patient's finances

Jay Malhotra, MD, Burr Ridge, IL

Eustacian: A London tube stop between T & V

Sidney Gold, MD, Woodland Hills, CA

Frank Pus: A great guy with an unusual last name.

Neal Green, MD, Corsicana, TX

Euthanasia: Children from the Far East

Anthony R. Russo, MD, Chesapeake, VA

Coup and contra-coup: Reagan's South American policy

David L. Taylor, MD, Oldsmar, FL

Autologous: Pertaining to a backseat driver

Jonathan S. Ehrlich, MD, Atlanta, GA

Masturbator: Professional fishing guide

Alton Romero, Jr., MD, Kaplan, LA

GREAT WORDS

ASSIGNMENT:
Provide a historical quote and its source, and give it a medical rationale.

EXAMPLES:
"Let them eat cake!" (Marie-Antoinette): Pronouncement on discovery of a cure for diabetes

"Nuts!" (General Anthony McAuliffe): Head of psychiatric facility's reason for resignation

"This is not the end. It is not even the beginning of the end . . . . But it is, perhaps, the end of the beginning." (Winston Churchill): Endoscopist, upon viewing the ascending colon

ENTRIES:
"Après nous, le déluge." (reply to Louis XV): Urologist about to relieve urinary obstruction

Ivan Safonoff, MD, Stockton, NJ

Bernadine Z. Paulshock, MD, Wilmington, DE

"What lies behind us and what lies before us are tiny matters compared to what lies within us." (Ralph Waldo Emerson): Obstetrician to patient suffering from hemorrhoids and a very big belly.

John Fox, MD, Richland, WA

"I shall return." (General Douglas MacArthur): What a dose of ipecac might say on its way down the esophagus.

John B. Parker, MD, Gig Harbor, WA

"More, more, more for labor." (Samuel Gompers): Calculating optimal dosage of labor-inducing drug.

Daniel J. Colombi, MD, Haddonfield, NJ

"I am alone with the masses." (Mao Tse-Tung): Unassisted surgeon doing emergency laparotomy in the wee hours, upon encountering multiple fibroids and ovarian cysts.

Tejinder S. Sandhu, MD, Sanger, CA

"Fourscore and seven years . . ." (Abraham Lincoln): Physician lamenting the time for insurance payment

Dave Taube, Eugene, OR

"They shall not pass." (Marshall Philippe Petain): Urologist regarding many large stones.

Mariano Villasenor, MD, Pittsburgh, PA

"What do you take me for, an idiot?" (General Charles de Gaulle): Hospital CEO, asked if he was happy.

Sivaprasad D. Madduri, MD, Poplar Bluff, MO

"Spare no expense to make everything as economical as possible (Samuel Goldwyn): From HMO medical director's newsletter to member physicians

Gregory Lee Smith, MD, Indianapolis, IN

"I only regret that I have but one life to give for my country." (Nathan Hale): Lymphocyte entering abscess cavity

Robert G. Allison, MD, Panorama City, CA

"There is no mistake; there has been no mistake; and there shall be no mistake." (Duke of Wellington): Defense attorney at negligence hearing

Alfred R. D'Angelo, MD, Ormond Beach, FL

"My specialty is being right when other people are wrong." (George Bernard Shaw): Pathologist at an M&M conference.

Anatoly Belilovsky, MD, Brooklyn, NY

"I'm not prone to argue." (Cleopatra): Patient to gynecologist

Richard K. Crissman, MD, Grand Rapids, MI

"Why don't you come up and see me sometime?" (Mae West): Patient requesting a house call

Stanley Mendelowitz, MD, Tarrytown, NY

"A penny saved is a penny earned." (Benjamin Franklin): HMO employee

Gerald Harris, MD, San Francisco, CA

MUSIC TO MY EARS

ASSIGNMENT:
Select a cell phone tune and match it to the caller's medical predicament.

EXAMPLES:
Eine kleine Nachtmusik: Sleep apnea
Dance of the Sugarplum Fairy: Unstable diabetes
Groove Is in the Heart: Saturday night trauma at the ER

ENTRIES:
Chopsticks: Bilateral leg fractures
Timothy Kutz, MD, Kutztown, PA

Falstaff Overture: Erectile dysfunction
Ethan Flaks, MD, Jamesville, NY

Hi Lilli, Hi Lo: Bipolar disorder
Meyer Hodes, MD, Far Rockaway, NY

We Got the Beat: Pacemaker dysfunction
Stephen Schulman, MD, Denton, TX

Wedding March: Acute cystitis
Bernadine Z. Paulshock, MD, Wilmington, DE

Whole Lotta Shakin' Goin' On: Epileptic Seizure
Ronald Olah, MD, Pasadena, CA

Carnaval des Animaux: DTs
Michael G. Mazur, MD, Rockford, IL

The Flight of the Bumble Bee: Tinnitus
Sham R. Bajina, MD, Woodbury, NJ

Mame: Farm equipment accident
Amy Porter, MD, La Canada, CA

Fire and Rain: Urinary tract infection
J. Miller, MD, Fairway, KS

A-B-C-D-E-F-G: Hepatitis
Anatoly Belilovsky, MD, Brooklyn, NY

Dance of the Hours: Insomnia
Sidney Gold, MD, Woodland Hills, CA

Song of the Volga Boatmen: Mother in labor
C. Dan Allen, MD, Atlanta, GA

My Eyes Are Fully Open: Graves' disease
Roy S. Goodman, MD, White Lake, MI

Rhapsody in Blue: Severe COPD
Rudi Kirschner, MD, Phoenix, AZ

Fascinatin' Rhythm: Abnormal EKG
Jim Sammon, MD, Springfield, MO

The Spinning Song: Vertigo
Russell J. Cox, MD, Gastonia, NC
Kimball R. Orton, MD, Tucson, AZ

The Rising: Priapism
Ira Kohn, MD, Clarks Summit, PA

The Wayward Wind: Intestinal hyperperistalsis
Mackenzie Smith, MD, Mercer Island, WA

Jingle Bells: Meniere's disease with tinnitus
D'nese M. Sokolowski, MD, Allentown, PA

Blue Moon: Green Bay Packer fan with frostbite from metal seat
Vincent Keipper, MD, Concord, NC

Looking For Love in all the Wrong Places: Patient in ophthalmology office with herpes of the eye.

L. Ralph Rogers, MD, Newburgh, IN

Nocturine: Prostatic hypertrophy

Ralph M. Kniseley, MD, Oak Ridge, TN

Love Is a Many-Splendored Thing: Herpes genitalis

John Lattin, MD, Fresno, CA

O Canada: Prescription refill request for Canadian Pharmacy

Linda Engstrom, RN, Concord, NC

AESCULAPIAN TALES

ASSIGNMENT:
Choose a name from your favorite fairy tale or nursery rhyme that lends itself to a job in the medical field.

EXAMPLES:
The Little Match Girl: Petite technician with big blood bank responsibility
Goldilocks: The one with the key to Medicare disbursement funds
Snow White and the Seven Dwarfs: Ethically pure endocrinologist with her pituitary research volunteers

ENTRIES:
Aladdin: Endoscopist who can see anywhere

Carol R. Porch, MD, Guntersville, AL

Cinderella: Black lung specialist

Floyd T. Nasuti, MD, Philadelphia, PA

Jabberwocky: HMO policy clarifier

Charles W. Webb, MD, Traverse City, MI

The Wizard of Oz: A very skilled colposcopist

Daniel J. Colombi, MD, Haddonfield, NJ

Princess and the Pea: Anorexic teenage girl

Robert Swietarski, MD, Westminster, CO

Goofy and Dopey: Co-authors of HIPAA regulations

Francis C. Bruno, MD, Columbia, MD

Cinderella: Lithotripsy technician

Glenn Lambert, MD, Flemington, NJ

Jack Horner: Ptotic pulmonary oncologist

Paul S. Denker, MD, Clearwater, FL

Twelve Dancing Princesses: King's daughters suffering from ADHD

Linda S. Woodson, MD, Las Vegas, NV

The Poor Man and the Rich Man: Family physician and cardiothoracic surgeon

Meyer Hodes, MD, Oceanside, NY

Paul Bunyan: Podiatrist to the NBA

Russell J. Cox, MD, Gastonia, NC

Wynken, Blynken, and Nod: Tic disorder specialists

Mackenzie Smith, MD, Mercer Island, WA

Uncle Remus: Urologist who performs TURPs

Dave Taube, Eugene, OR

Jack Spratt: Poster child for bariatric surgery

Allan LaReau, MD, Kalamazoo, MI

The cow that jumped over the moon: Lab animal in steroid research

Neal Green, MD, Corsicana, TX

The Big Bad Wolf: The most despised malpractice lawyer in town

Douglas Clark, MD, Seattle, WA

The Good Fairy: The one person at the HMO you could count on to OK your claims; who one day waved her magic wand and, "POOF," disappeared

Stanley Rogers, DO, Oklahoma City, OK

Sleeping Beauty: CPAP success

Anthony R. Russo, MD, Chesapeake, VA

Three Little Pigs: CEO, CFO, COO, of HMO

Multiple contributors

Rumpelstiltskin: A tall geriatric dermatologist

Vincent Keipper, MD, Concord, NC

Humpty Dumpty: Typical ER "Saturday Night Special"

Allan B. Solum, MD, Paynesville, MN

TAG, YOU'RE IT

ASSIGNMENT:
Luggage pieces being similar, how may a specialist make his/her bag identifiable at the baggage claim?

EXAMPLES:
Ophthalmologist: Attached Snellen eye chart reading THISISMYBAG
Obstetrician: Bag undergoes periodic contractions
Laparoscopist: Each surface of the luggage has three portholes

ENTRIES:
Neonatologist: A bag weighing only one pound, fourteen ounces
Neal Green, MD, Corsicana, TX

Geneticist: Double-helix-shaped luggage
Daniel J. Colombi, MD, Haddonfield, NJ

A dozen specialists: One outsized bag labeled RISK POOL
John Lattin, MD, Fresno, CA

Pulmonologist: Bag is normally blue but turns pink when met with oxygen
Kathy Waller, MD, Ft. Collins, CO

Geriatrician: Old, weathered suitcase on a walker instead of a roller
Scott Crawford, MD, Phoenix, AZ

HMO gatekeeper: Bag has little hidden springs that bump it off the luggage carousel after a few minutes
Alan L. Goldman, MD, Raleigh, NC

Otologist: Bag beeps at various frequencies until identified by owner
Marina Claudio, MD, Chicago, IL

Coroner: Bag has toe tag instead of a luggage tag.
Steven Preston, MD, Elizabethtown, KY

Neurologist: Unobtrusive bag twitches and shouts expletives

Lisa Shakerin, MD, Robbinsdale, MN

Cardiologist: Bag pulsates and emits sounds at normal sinus rhythm.

Bernadine Z. Paulshock, MD, Wilmington, DE

Rheumatologist: Handle can retract only partly, shaft being slightly bent

Wade Anderson, MD, Fairmont, MN

Urologist: Foley catheter instead of ribbon on handle

Britt Smith, MD, Olympia, WA

Obstetrician: Luggage is tied up with an umbilical cord.

Robert Edelman, MD, Mill Neck, NY

Endocrinologist: Set made up of largest and smallest bags on conveyor

Alfred R. D'Angelo, MD, Ormond Beach, FL

Family physician: Well-worn trunk with a dozen handles, covered in souvenir stickers from ICU, office, patients' homes, etc.

Cynthia G. Olsen, MD, Yellow Springs, OH

HEEL COOLING

ASSIGNMENT:
For "Waiting Room," substitute "Welcome, please have a seat in the ___, and the ___ will be with you shortly." Then fill in the blanks with an appropriate name for the antechamber and the corresponding practitioner.

EXAMPLES:
Scrotunda/urologist
Secrete passageway/endocrinologist
Solarium/podiatrist

ENTRIES:
Tacky atrium/electrophysiologist

> Wynnshang Sun, MD, La Jolla, CA

Cloac room/proctologist

> William Ameen, MD, Greensboro, NC

Antecubicle/phlebotomist

> Allan B. Solum, MD, Paynesville, MN

Bored room/chronically late physician

> Russell J. Cox, MD, Gastonia, NC

Rantechamber/psychotherapist

> Laura Donegan, MD, Laurel, MD

Lesser space/surgeon

> Meyer Hodes, MD, Oceanside, NY

Cell block/pathologist

> A. E. Mgebroff, MD, Yoakum, TX

Fitting room/neurologist

> Michael C. Joseph, MD, Baltimore, MD

Courtyard/high-risk obstetrician
Joseph F. J. Curi, MD, Torrington, CT

Control room/robotic surgeon
Richard L. Julius, MD, St. Petersburg, FL

Discotheque/orthopedist
Don Allen, MD, Atlanta, GA

Dead space/pulmonologist
Michael J. Crook, MD, Glens Falls, NY

Vasilica/urologist
Samir B. G. Boutros, MD, South Hill, VA

Corncrib/podiatrist
Alfred R. D'Angelo, DO, Ormond Beach, FL

Altar/transgender surgeon
Glenn Perelson, MD, Chula Vista, CA

Grand ballroom/urologist
Ivan Safonoff, MD, Stockton, NJ

Hippo campus/neurologist or liposuctionist (shared office)
Daniel Schual-Berke, Seattle, WA
Similarly (Hippodrome), Jeff Lenow, MD,
Medford, NJ

Drawing room/hematologist
E. Gallenstein, MD, Cincinnati, OH

Callouseum/podiatrist
Allan Plaut, MD, Lawrence, NY

Wreck room/trauma surgeon
Kathleen L. Norton, MD, Omaha, NE

Rectory/proctologist
James D. Garrity, MD, Monroe, CT

Drop zone/obstetrician

Jeffrey L. Lenow, MD, Medford, NJ

Holding tank/urologist

Dan Mackey, MD, Santa Ana, CA

Breezeway/pulmonologist

Aletha Oglesby, MD, Tulsa, OK

Pullpit/pediatric ER physician

Glenn Perelson, MD, Chula Vista, CA

AND THAT'S AN ORDER!

ASSIGNMENT:
Alter a well-known exhortation into a medical command or motto.

EXAMPLES:
Make love, not spore! (Avoid yeast infections!)
Grime does not pay! (Scrub for the required time!)
Don't give up the scrip! (Go easy on OTC medicines!)
Keep on trochin'! (Remember the power of throat lozenges!)

ENTRIES:
Don't worry, be HIPAA! (Enjoy your own Notice of Privacy Practices!)
Lisa Shakerin, MD, Robbinsdale, MN

Remember the a la mode! (Stick to your diet!)
G. J. Billmeier, Jr., MD, Memphis, TN

Take it wheezy! (Use your inhaler as needed!)
Wade Anderson, MD, Fairmont, MN

Go for the mold! (Utilize Olympic antifungal agent!)
Melvin J. Breite, MD, Bayside, NY

Send in the crowns! (Advice for dental assistants)
Herbert Gersh, MD, Treasure Island, FL

Take me to your bleeder! (We're the EMs, we're here, so use us!)
Ivan Safonoff, MD, Stockton, NJ

Go test, young man! (Invest in an office lab!)
Meyer Hodes, MD, Oceanside, NY
Similarly, J. R. Mehta, MD, Los Angeles, CA

Damn the turbinates; full speed ahead! (Nasopharyngoscopy)
David Gould, MD, Houston, TX

Cram the torpedoes! (Use all the suppositories!)

Richard K. Crissman, MD, Grand Rapids, MI

Damn the placebos! Full speed ahead! (We don't need a controlled study!)

Michael Ichniowski, MD, Lutherville, MD

Don't give up the shape! (Bariatrician's advice)

Bernadine Z. Paulshock, MD, Wilmington, DE

Never say sever! (You can save that foot!)

Irving Thorne, MD, Minneapolis, MN

One strep at a time! (Don't get overwhelmed in the pediatric clinic!)

Vincent Keipper, MD, Concord, NC

Let them be light! (Don't allow the kids to eat junk food and supersize!)

Lyn S. Aye, MD, Auburn, CA

Powder to the people! (Keep that skin dry!)

Daniel J. Colombi, MD, Haddonfield, NJ

Ask not what your country can do for sprue, ask what it can do for your country! (Avoid glutens!)

David Taube, MD, Eugene, OR

One good sperm deserves another! (Re-donate to your local fertility clinic today!)

James A. Shubin, MD, Sebastopol, CA

Everything's coming up noses! (Steroid nasal spray's the thing for you!)

Gene E. Ress, MD, Tell City, IN

PLAYING WITH WORDS

ASSIGNMENT:
Words and phrases often convey double meanings. Apply this to medical conversation.

EXAMPLES:
What's new under the sun in skin cancer?
What's going down in swallowing disorders?
They went with the flow at the urology convention.
Cryogenics is the tip of the therapeutic iceberg.

ENTRIES:
Finding no Y chromosomes, the geneticist knew something was a-miss.

Scott Crawford, MD, Phoenix, AZ

Give me the lowdown on achondroplasia.

Steven Preston, MD, Elizabethtown, KY

The man who had a hemicorporectomy is all right now.

Mitchell A. Kopnick, MD, Janesville, WI

What's the story with Munchausen's syndrome?

Jesse Hackell, MD, Pomona, NY

The surgeon doing the sex-change operation had his patient asleep at the switch.

K. C. Price, MD/M. B. Price, RN, Gonzales, TX

A ventriculoperitoneal shunt is a real brain drain.

Ike Koziol, MD, Manakin-Sabot, VA

Ambidextrous patients are sometimes gauche.

Myron Siner, MD, Wellesley, MA

Dextrocardia means having your heart in the right place.

Joseph Grayzel, MD, Englewood, NJ

Was the urologist's paper peer reviewed?

Leonard V. Fisher, MD, Los Angeles, CA

The infectious disease consultant appreciates his staff.

Michael J. Mutchler, MD, Hubbardston, MA

How sweet it is to reverse an insulin reaction.

Joseph F. J. Curi, MD, Torrington, CT

The ophthalmology professor had a keen eye for good pupils.

Michael J. Crook, MD, Glens Falls, NY

"That's what happens when the rubber meets the road," explained the STD physician.

Richard K. Crissman, MD, Grand Rapids, MI

When it comes to hearing, otology is the whole ball of wax.

Dave Taube, MD, Eugene, OR

You gotta know when to hold 'em in urology.

Daniel J. Colombi, MD, Haddonfield, NJ

Treatment for a kleptomaniac: Give him something to take.

Adon S. Weinberg, DO, Youngstown, OH

Genetics is just a twist of nature.

Michael Markoff, MD, Red Bank, NJ

The obese consult dietitians to reduce a problem of increasing gravity.

Newton G. Osborne, MD, Bethesda, MD

Intubation is like a breath of fresh air.

June Melin, MD, San Diego, CA

FUNNY BONE

ASSIGNMENT:
Choose a comic strip or cartoon character, alter the name (if need be), and describe the character's new medical profession.

EXAMPLES:
Hegar the Horrible: Infamous gynecologist
Dick Bracy: Orthotics merchant
Tweezix: Microsurgeon of Gasoline Alley
Little Endorphin Annie: Neurotransmitter authority

ENTRIES:
For Butter or for Wurst: A lipid doctor's nightmare
Herbert Gersh, MD, Treasure Island, FL

Finding Chemo: The runaway oncologist
Glenn S. Sherman, MD, Allentown, PA

The Little Spermaid: Infertility technologist
Anne E. Walker, MD, Charlotte, NC

Suey, Hooey, and Phooey: Malpractice lawyers
Melvin Breite, MD, Bayside, NY

Spayderman: Pregnancy prevention specialist
Alan L. Goldman, MD, Raleigh, NC

Captain Marbles: Psychiatrist
Richard L. Julius, MD, St. Petersburg, FL

Hot Flash Gordon: Menopause expert
Daniel J. Colombi, MD, Haddonfield, NJ

The Born Loser: Solo, fee-for-service practitioner
Eric Strauss, MD, Portola Valley, CA

Gasper: The friendly pulmonologist

Steven Preston, MD, Elizabethtown, KY

Snoopy: Utilization reviewer

David P. Perkins, MD, St. Davids, PA

Flex Morgan, MD: Endoscopist

O. Scott Lauter, MD, Lancaster, PA

The Green Goblet: Sinister sinusitis specialist

Jeffrey L. Lenow, MD, Medford, NJ

Charley Brown-Sequard: Athletically challenged spinal cord specialist

Gilbert Herzberg, MD, New York, NY

Blandie: Dated gastroenterologist

Alfred D'Angelo, DO, Ormond Beach, CA

Peanuts: Urologist who treats hypoplastic gonads by day and works as an HMO paymaster by night

Richard K. Crissman, MD, Grand Rapids, MI

Hepar the Horrible: Liver transplant surgeon owning bourbon distillery

Sham R. Bajina, MD, Woodbury, NJ

Needle Bailey: Acupuncturist

Allan B. Solum, MD, Paynesville, MN

Fatman and the Incredible Hulk: Bariatric surgical group

C. D. Allen, MD, Atlanta, GA

AFTERNOON T

ASSIGNMENT:
Conceive of a T-shirt message worn by the appropriate specialist.

EXAMPLES:
Dermatologist: I started from scratch.

Cardiologist: I went to a cardiology seminar and all I got was this lousy pqrsT-shirt!

Surgeon: This T-shirt was a cardigan prior to the stapling.

ENTRIES:
Gastroenterologist: E Pluribus Jejunum
<blockquote>Daniel J. Colombi, MD, Haddonfield, NJ</blockquote>

Parasitologist: I went to work today and all I got was this louse-y T-shirt.
<blockquote>Mark Greenfield, MD, Seattle, WA</blockquote>

Psychiatrist: You think, therefore I am.
<blockquote>Aletha Oglesby, MD, Tulsa, OK</blockquote>

Urologist: Meyer's Toolworks. Yours can too!
<blockquote>Meyer Hodes, MD, Oceanside, NY</blockquote>

Surgeon: As ye sew, dough shall ye reap.
<blockquote>Tom Savoie, MD, Elkhart, IN</blockquote>

Obstetrician: Push, push, Sweet Charlotte
<blockquote>Julio C. Novoa, MD, Perry Hall, MD</blockquote>

Chief of cardiology: I'm the cor corps core.
<blockquote>Ivan Safonoff, MD, Stockton, NJ</blockquote>

Neurologist: The wearer of this shirt axon impulses.
<blockquote>Dave Taube, MD, Eugene, OR</blockquote>

Nephrologist: I am proud of my Peer group.
<blockquote>Peter A. Noronha, MD, Oak Brook, IL</blockquote>

Plastic surgeon: Objects may appear larger after surgery.

Michael T. McNamara, MD, High Point, NC

Gyn: I'M IN PR—PELVIC RELATIONS.

Barry Kramer, MD, Los Angeles, CA

Podiatrist: Who wants to marry a bunionaire?

Don Murrmann, MD, Kerrville, TX

Geneticist: GENETICISTS MAKE BETTER LOVERS. Can we make you one?

David P. Perkins, MD, St. Davids, PA

Urologist: I (heart symbol) the Rolling Stones.

Joseph Grayzel, MD, Englewood, NJ

Cardiologist: V1, V2 . . . V6 in anatomically correct positions

Anatoly Belilovsky, MD, Brooklyn, NY

Radiologist: Need a PET? Try a CAT.

Timothy Kutz, MD, Kutztown, PA

Ophthalmologist: I doctor!

Debbi Silverman, MD, Cincinnati, OH

Ophthalmologist: If you can read this, you don't need to be here.

Michael Illingworth, MD, Clovis, CA

Proctologist: Business is looking up!

Joseph T. Gromada, MD, Cincinnati, OH

YOU CALL THIS MEDICAL NEWS?

ASSIGNMENT:
Create a provocative headline that appears to be of medical interest until the subheadline and subsequent story show how the reader was misled.

EXAMPLES:
SIAMESE TWINS, JOINED AT THE HEAD, SEPARATED: Thai sibling sailors forced to use different shipboard facilities.

CALCULUS PASSED BY CEO'S SON: After months of tutoring, boy finally gets a 65 in math.

ENTRIES:
LO FAT VERY DANGEROUS: Notorious Chinese gang leader suspected in wave of violence.

Frank Bruno, MD, Columbia, MD

BYPASS FAILS TO RESTORE FLOW AFTER MI: Pavement buckle snarls highway detour traffic out of Ann Arbor.

Mitchell A. Kopnick, MD, Janesville, WI

GIANT CELL REACTION CAUSED BY LOCAL IRRITANT: Huge number of cell phone customers complain of local business's annoying telemarketing practices.

Andrew Malinchak, DO, Covington, GA

SMOKING SHOWN TO PROLONG LIFE SPAN: Salmon now lasts up to four months on shelf.

Steven Preston, MD, Elizabethtown, KY

TUBE FEEDING DISCONTINUED: Food no longer allowed on London Underground.

Ron Jones, MD, Nevada, MO

RIBS REMOVED WITHOUT CONSENT: Police investigate barbecue eatery break-in.

Neal Green, MD, Corsicana, TX

LIMB REPLACEMENT APPEARS SUCCESSFUL: Local tree surgeon grafts apple branch to peach tree.

Richard K. Crissman, MD, Grand Rapids, MI

MORE DOCTORS CHOOSING CT FOR JOINT EVALUATION: Connecticut found to be prime setting for study of marijuana's effects.

Tom Savoie, MD, Elkhart, IN

COLON FUNCTION DEEMED REGULAR NATIONWIDE: English language scholar explains correct usage of punctuation marks.

Meyer Hodes, MD, Oceanside, NY

SEIZURE LEAVES MAN CRIPPLED: Illegal weapons confiscation cripples criminal's case.

Robert E. Resnick, MD, JD, Oceanside, NY

HEARTS STOLEN FROM LOCAL HOSPITAL: Thieves walk away with Valentine candy from gift shop.

Russell J. Cox, MD, Gastonia, NC

FAT DEPOSITS PROVE BENEFICIAL: Bank declares dividend.

Richard L. Julius, MD, St. Petersburg, FL

MAYOR SHOT: City CEO first to receive flu vaccine.

Morey Filler, MD, San Francisco, CA

EGGS RETRIEVED FROM SEVENTY-FIVE-YEAR-OLD DONOR: Local Boy Scout troop collects eggs from farmer for benefit breakfast.

Stephen Brown, MD, Marcellus, NY

ODDS AT 20 TO 1 FOR INHERITING SKIN CANCER: Inheriting Skin Cancer is long shot at racetrack this weekend.

Nancy Guttman, MD, Augusta, KY

BETA BLOCKADE PREVENTS ERECTION: Beta Theta brothers gather to prevent erection of rival fraternity Gamma Delta homecoming tent . . .

Melvin J. Breite, MD, Bayside, NY

THE TRICENTENNIAL (300th contest)

ASSIGNMENT:
Create a medical situation involving the number 300.

EXAMPLES:
Fertility specialist: "With a sperm count like this, it will take a star in the East."

Internist: "Gotta get that cholesterol down a mite."

Bariatrician: "Be it pounds or kilos, this is morbid."

ENTRIES:
Pediatrician: I know those triplets are sick, but I wish their mom would give me the temperatures separately!

Alan L. Goldman, MD, Raleigh, NC

Urologist: If he can count to 300 while trying to empty, he'd better consult me.

Richard L. Julius, MD, St. Petersburg, FL

Urologist: You took 300 tablets instead of a 300 mg. tablet for ED?

Morey Filler, MD, San Francisco, CA

Sports medicine specialist: With a platelet count like this, I would call for a fair catch.

Joseph F. J. Curi, MD, Torrington, CT

Gerontologist: You don't look a day older than 299.

Dave Taube, MD, Eugene, OR

Family physician: Didn't you know that was a beehive?

Meyer Hodes, MD, Oceanside, NY

Surgeon: 300 sutures and the wound still puckers?

Hugh H. Wang, MD, Pleasant Hill, CA

Obstetrician: Gravida-300, para-lyzed!

Suzanne Dixson, MD, Fort Worth, TX

Podiatrist: 300 is a nice number of feet for a football field, or for 150 podiatrists.

Neal Green, MD, Corsicana, TX

Sleep specialist: 300 sheep is just not enough for a diagnosis of insomnia.

Helen S. Percy, MD, Lahaina, HI

Pediatrician: Worst case of polydactyly I've ever seen!

Gene Westveer, MD, Zeeland, MI

Family physician: Congratulations! You're the 300th patient, so your visit is free, aside from the $300 co-pay.

Stephen L. Kaufman, MD, San Francisco, CA

Geneticist: Wow, you win this week's café-au-lait contest!

Amy Porter, MD, La Canada, CA

Ophthalmologist: 20/300 in each eye? Maybe we should just drive locally.

Melvin J. Breite, MD, Bayside, NY

Pharmacist: Yes, per month. But only with the new Medicare drug card.

Eric Strauss, MD, Portola Valley, CA

Nephrologist: With a BUN like that, we'll need a triuretic.

Steven Preston, MD, Elizabethtown, KY

Psychologist: With an IQ like this, I'd like to discuss a few of my problems with you.

Richard Walters, MD, Webster Groves, MO

Family physician: We've got to talk to the new girl about the scheduling!

Alfred R. D'Angelo, DO, Ormond Beach, FL

Internist: Your 300 weight, cholesterol, triglycerides, blood sugar and blood pressure are not the kind of equality Jefferson had in mind.

Ivan Safonoff, MD, Stockton, NJ

BEEPLESS IN SEATTLE (AND ELSEWHERE)

ASSIGNMENT:

In reaching voice mail, a beep invites you to leave a message. Suppose the recorded voice invites you to do so after a more appropriate sound? Conceive of one.

EXAMPLES:

GERD specialist: "Please leave your message after the sound of the burp."
Urologist: "Please wait for the deep sigh of relief, then leave your message."
Psychiatrist: "Leave your message after the creak of the couch springs."

ENTRIES:

Psychiatrist: "If you're a paranoid schizophrenic, there is no need to leave a message, since we know who you are and why you've called."

Anthony Russo, MD, Chesapeake, VA

Clinic administrator: "Leave a message after the co-pay is deposited." (Hear coins dropping into a can.)

Russell J. Cox, MD, Gastonia, NC

Sex therapist: "Leave no message. Instead, contact me via my Web site: sextherapy.org.org.org."

Leland Whitson, MD, Redondo Beach, CA

Pre-cert nurse: "Leave your request and then press 1 to hear a snicker, 2 for a chortle, or 3 for a guffaw."

Stanley Hartness, MD, Kosciusko, MS

Transplant surgeon: "Leave a message at the sound of the organ."

Thomas McGrath, MD, Storrs, CT

Bariatrician: "All lines are busy. We're sorry for your weight. Press the pound sign and begin."

William C. Cartmill, MD, Paw Paw, MI

Obstetrician: "Leave your message after the beep and push! push! push! any button when finished."

Neal Green, MD, Corsicana, TX

Hematologist: "Leave a message of any type."

Richard E. Behymer, MD, Sonora, CA

Sleep specialist: "When the snoring stops, you'll have twenty seconds to leave a message before it starts again."

Gene Westveer, MD, Zeeland, MI

Cardiologist: "Please leave your murmurs after the click."

Kirk Muffly, MD, Omaha, NE

Research lab: "When the dogs stop barking, leave your message."

Bernadine Z. Paulshock, MD, Wilmington, DE

HMO clinic: "Please leave your message after the gate clangs shut, even though we won't get back to you."

Ronald Olah, MD, Pasadena, CA

Hypnotherapist: "When I snap my fingers, you will leave a message!"

Alfred R. D'Angelo, MD, Ormond Beach, FL

Audiologist: "Record your message after the glockenspiel."

Joseph F. J. Curi, MD, Torrington, CT

HAVE AN UNBAD DAY

ASSIGNMENT:
Modify the hackneyed "Have a good day" according to specialty.

EXAMPLES:
Pediatrician: Have a day that will live in infancy.
Gastroenterologist: Have a comme cecum ça day.
Urologist: May your day flow with serenity.

ENTRIES:
Managed-care functionary: Have a good yesterday. We're not paying for today.

Melvin J. Breite, MD, Bayside, NY

Infectious disease specialist: May profuse growth of positive experiences fill your plate today.

Graciano L. Zara, MD, North Brunswick, NJ

Surgeon to reconnected colostomy patient: May the wind be always at your back.

Don Chiles, MD, Fullerton, CA

Utilization reviewer: Have a day—that's all your DRG allows

Steven Preston, MD, Elizabethtown, KY

Fluid/electrolyte specialist: Have a normal day.

Alan L. Goldman, MD, Raleigh, NC

Alternative medicine physician: Have a good thyme.

Allan LaReau, MD, Kalamazoo, MI

Capitated GP: May you stay healthy and never come back.

James Ulery, Jr., MD, Monroe, WI

Impotence specialist: Have a very hard day.

Daniel J. Colombi, MD, Haddonfield, NJ

Anesthesiologist: Happy daze.

Bernadine Z. Paulshock, MD, Wilmington, DE

Speech pathologist: Have a dice nay.

Morey Filler, MD, San Francisco, CA

Pulmonologist: May you have great expectorations.

Alfred D'Angelo, DO, Ormond Beach, FL

Intensivist: I will C that U have a nice day.

Andrew Malinchak, DO, Covington, GA

Obstetrician: Push your day to a crowned happiness.

Julio C. Novoa, MD, Perry Hall, MD

Surgeon: Suture self to a wonderful day.

Morton Krieger, MD, Baltimore, MD

VITAL TITLES

ASSIGNMENT:
Medically alter the title of a poem. Briefly explain its new meaning.

EXAMPLES:
"The Ream of the Ancient Mariner": TUR in a naval hospital

"Do Not Go Dental into That Good Night": Make sure to choose medical school.

"Jabberwacky": Tale of an overzealous phlebotomist

"Fra Lippo Lippy": A monk who does facial surgery

ENTRIES:
"Uvulume": Edgar Allan Poe's laryngoscope

Evelyn Weissman, MD, Malone, NY

"How Do I Glove Me?": Protecting me from thee and thee from me

Hugh Wang, MD, Concord, CA

"The Shaven": After a craniotomy, patient tells his neurosurgeon, "Nevermore."

Steven Schulman, MD, Denton, TX

"Sí, Fever": Latino patient's answer to his doctor's first question.

Alan L. Goldman, MD, Raleigh, NC

"I Wandered Lonely as a Clot": A coagulation looking for a place to attach itself

Dave Taube, MD, Solar Heights, OR

"Ben Dover Beach": Facility known for its top-notch prostate surveillance

David Perkins, MD, St. David's PA

"Past Midnight Ride of Paul Revere": Looking for an ER that accepts your insurance

Morey Filler, MD, San Francisco, CA

"Ode on a Grecian Urinal": Urology patient on Aegean tour
P. Schlein, MD, Richmond, VA

"A Man's a Woman for A' That": Tome on sex-change surgery
Ron Jones, MD, Nevada, MO

"When We Two Parted": Conjoined twins, post-op
Herb Gersh, MD, Treasure Island, FL

"On First Looking into Chapman's Tumor": Classic oncologic staging
Daniel Colombi, MD, Haddonfield, NJ

"Leda and the Swan-Ganz": Drama in the cardiac cath lab
Russell J. Cox, MD, Gastonia, NC

"The Clod and the Pebble": Maladroit urologist attempting lithotripsy
Lyn Aye, MD, Auburn, CA

ON THE RIBALD SIDE

During the life of the Wits End series, a number of submissions ranging from R- to X-rated made their way into the mass of entries. It was felt best not to publish them lest an avalanche of bawdiness invade the propriety of the contests. They were, however, saved. For the sake of completeness in re the craft of creativity, these earthy contributions herewith see the light of day. They are listed according to the titles of the contests in which they appeared. The authors are anonymous. For all we know, some may want it that way.

O GIVE ME A HOME
    Sexologist—French Lick, IN
    Proctologist—South Bendover, IN (FC)

SPECIALTY OF THE HOUSE
    Urologist—The Cock and Bull
    Sexologist—Phallus's Restaurant (Cervix with a Smile)

SPORTS MEDICINE
    The Cremasters—Players noted for ball control
    The Priapisms—"We're up for every game!"

THE FIRING LINE
    Gynecologist—Screwed/laid off
    Urologist—Pissed off/discharged
    Proctologist—Assassinated

IN SITU
    Sag Harbor—Clinic for impotent seamen
    Bangkok—Penile prosthetic field testing lab
    Bangkok—Home of renowned penile trauma center
    Mount Comfort, IN—Dyspareunia treatment center
    Athol, MA—Proctologic capital of the world
    Coxsackie—Scrotal support manufacturing

SLOGAN'S HEROES
    Penile implant surgeon—It's what's up front that counts.

RUSSIAN DRESSINGS
Beware the reckless Russian urologist I. Kutchapeckeroff

UNINITIATION RITES
Carcinogen—Sexual activity resulting in the birth of talk show hosts

POLITICAL PARADOX
My opponent is hard on impotence.

IT SPEAKS VOLUMES
Question: Do you have a book on impotence?
Answer: Only in soft cover.

Q: . . . premature ejaculation?
A: Yes, but you can only check it out for thirty seconds.

Q: . . . sadism/masochism?
A: At the binder, being bound—in leather.

Q: . . . nymphomaniacal disorders?
A: Can't get enough of them!

Q: . . . urinary urgency?
A: It's out. You'll have to get a hold on it.

Q: . . . multiple orgasms?
A: Fiction.

Q: . . . impotence?
A: Yes, it's in the basement stacks. We're having trouble getting it up.

Q: . . . erectile dysfunction?
A: Yes, they're coming up slowly.

SAY IT AGAIN, SAM
Urologist Sebastian Chamfort providing a literary criticism on a
  couplet: "Excellent, were it not for its length."
Mae West, sex therapist: "Nice guys finish last."

HAVING HAD IT
Impotency therapist: Flaccid and unable to rise to the occasion

ACTA OPERATICA
Midsummer Night's Scream: About a faked orgasm
Taming of the Screw: Kate slows down Petruchio's quickies.

ER TO THE FAMOUS
"Mr. Queeg, we appreciate your allergic reaction to strawberries, but would you stop playing with your balls?"

MALAPROPERLY SPEAKING
(A true one): "My child went to a birthday party and caught a cocksucker-bee infection."
Honey, STD is no problem—I have a condominium.
On Her Majesty's cervix.

CLINICAL TRIAL
"Be certain; this is a hung jury," counseled the sex therapist.
"I'm responsible for that hung jury," the urologist bragged.
"All rise," intoned the penile implant surgeon.
"We have a hung jury," said the female urologist in measured tones.
THE SHORES OF TIPPLE-Y
The Pleasure Triangle—gynecologist
Lawrence of the Labia Lounge—gynecologist

MEMOIRS
David Cop-a-Feel—If a certain scandalized senator had been a physician . . . .
Mopey Dick—Infertility specialist
Lord of the Flies—Urologist
Goldfinger—Park Avenue gynecologist
Morbid Dick—Forensic pathologist

NOT QUITE TRITE
Do it lickety-split—Aberrant sex therapist
Never up, never in—Impotence
Hold your own—Onanism

IN A WORD

"Tamponade," replied the little vampire when asked to name his favorite beverage.

Vulvovaginitis—Why Swedes love their station wagons

"Diverticulum!"—What one snorkler instructed another complaining of scrotal itch

CALL WAITING

Penile prosthetist: *Rat-a-tat-tat* of woodpecker

Impotence specialist: Cock-a-doodle-doo

Sex therapist: Beeper keeps going off before the page

GAFFES À LA WEBB

He had a trick of Mona's infection . . . but his wife's name is Shirley.

Hospital building fund slogan: I upped my pledge—Up yours. (Now that's what I call a hard sell).

AT THE BRINK

Gynecologist (doing a Pap on a Giant Amazon): Tie the rope around my ankles now, and hold tight. I'm going in!

HANG YOUR HAT

Cystoscopist: Dixie Throughway

SPELL CHECK

Pseudomonas—Nonorgasmic

Smallcox—Microgenitalia

Striptococcus—Male exotic dance club

MATING SEASON

Allergist: A single prick looking for a positive response

Urologist specializing in impotence, seeking receptive female, would like to get something straight between us

DUPLEX

OB-GYN: Catch and snatch

WORD CONVERSION
Hospice: Where Premarin comes from

JOX TO DOX
Pete Rose: Viagra success story

PROVERBIAL SECOND CHANCE
Abstinence makes the frond grow harder.

TOOLING AROUND
Stopcock: Planned Parenthood at a poultry farm

AUTOMOBILITY
Everyone knows that the OB-GYN drives a Vulva, but when he gets
up in the world he switches to a Le Mons.
Grand Prix—Urologist

WITSENDER'S BRAIN
Casanova's wrist—A Viagra user who was stood up

SQUARE FOOTERS
Sashaying up and down the aisles
Hold her butt if she has piles.

DIAGNOSIS CONFIRMED
Victims that have fallen from the Firemen's Memorial in San Francisco:
Coitus interruptus

SKIN DEEP
Peter Patch: Transdermal Viagra

AUTHOR AND OPUS
Honore de Balsack: Testicular surgery in a nutshell

DRAMATIS PERSONAE
Hymen: A guardian of the Gates of Heaven

WELCOME MAT
Sperm donor suite: We'll have you coming and going in no time.
Come on in . . . a little.

ENTITLEMENT
Moby Dick: Impotent whale
Sea captain's priapism
Ball Four: Hypertestosteronism

THE CLINICAL TEAM
Trojans: Family planning specialists

WHAT WAS THAT YOU SAID?
Liposuction: A form of foreplay
Dick Test: Urologic short-arm inspection

MUSIC TO MY EARS
The Merry Wives of Windsor: Priapism
"Long Time Coming": Erectile dysfunction
"A Hard Day's Night": Priapism
"I Can't Get Started With You": Erectile dysfunction
"Don't Let Me Down"; "Come together": Viagra patient

AESCULAPIAN TALES
Peter Pan: Medical engineer, designer of sperm donor receptacles

AND THAT'S AN ORDER
Come out with your glans up—Viagra ad

FUNNY BONE
Fleanuts: Steroid abuse specialist, delayed adolescence endocrinologist, orchiopexist
Woody Woodpecker: Viagra detail man, urologist with mahogany implant technique
Dick Bracy: New erectile dysfunction product

Printed in the United States
146290LV00003B/15/P

9 781436 306157